Dear Darling Mike,
Keep on following
the Rainbows. Pot
of gold is in our
hearts!
♡
Love to you
Dr D.

Testimonials

Dr. D. Bluefish has been my chiropractor for over ten years. As a singer, songwriter, I travel the world, and Dr. D. is the BEST!

Colbie Callait

The moment you walk into the door, of the office, of Dr. D. Blue Fish, you feel cared for in every way! Dr. D. is highly intuitive, extremely knowledgeable and skillful in her work, AND she has a pair of extraordinary healing hands! You cannot help but trust Dr. D implicitly. When you walk out the door there is a sense of inner peace, health and well being at all levels. Everyone LOVES DR. D!

Lisa Luckenbach,

As a fashion designer, I travel on and off planes, trains and automobiles, am under constant stressful work situations and impossible deadlines. I have been to "the best" chiropractors in every city I travel to, LA, Beverly Hills, NYC, Milano, Paris, and Sydney, to name a few. Frustrated with the results I actually contemplated having Dr. D. come travel with me. NO ONE compares.

As a natural born healer, Dr. D is truly the only one who can put me back together, mentally and physically!

Sara Johnson

Dr. D. Bluefish, has been my chiropractor for 20 years, and has seen me through car accidents, falls, dislocation, torn ligaments, and even a spider bite in a "sensitive" area. Dr D's' holistic approach to well being, care and competence has put me back together every time. Her knowledgeable application of chiropractic, massage, and physical therapy has put me back on the road to recovery and mobility. I highly recommend Dr D. She is the best there is.

Nancy Martinez

Dr. D. has been my family's chiropractor for twenty years. She puts us back in alignment and before leaving her office, she gives us exercises and recommendations.   I recommend her to   all my friends and acquaintances and always get a hearty thank you.

Dale Hanson

At sixty seven years old, I have suffered from migraines, since I was eighteen. Until I found Dr. D., I have had to spend hours sleeping them off with the use of drugs. Through her wealth of knowledge, intuitive touch and years of experience, she has been able to alleviate the symptoms within an hour. Miraculous!

Darien Dragee

The Freak in the Grotto
True Stories to Help You Heal
by
<u>Dr. D. Blue Fish, BS, DC.</u>

Disclaimer

The purpose of this book is to provide entertainment. Through stories and essays, I present paths to self help and self healing. None of the recommendations in this book are to be used without first consulting a medical professional about any serious problem or condition. The author cannot accept any responsibility for errors or omissions or for any consequence from application of the information provided and makes no warranty, expressed or implied, with respect to the information provided. Thank You.

The stories presented in this book are based on true life stories and interactions with real patients. All names and particulars have been changed to protect their privacy. In every case, permission to print has been granted by the patients. Any resemblance these stories may have to anyone else is purely coincidental.

The Freak in the Grotto

True Stories to Help You Heal

By

Dr. D. Blue Fish, BS, DC

Introduction

Welcome to my world, where things aren't always what they seem. These stories, that I share with you, represent a portion of my practice, where pain originates, not with physical exertion, but with emotional turmoil. I offer these interesting stories of truth and consequences, as a guide to help others, who may be struggling with the same or similar problems.

Emotions can kill you.

Everyone is different and we all react differently to the hurdles that we face in life. One person may have no problem with their mother calling on the phone, and another will tweak their neck when they hear her voice. A brother dying, a spouse leaving the home, or a childhood drama that plays over and over again in your head, can cause true physical pain, even though, the true, root cause of the pain, originates in the psyche.

I like to think that I'm like *Felix the Cat,* I use every trick in my bag to help people heal. I might hold a metaphorical mirror up to their faces, hoping to guide them through the darkness into the light, helping them to discover and process the hidden cause of their symptoms. I, wholeheartedly, dig into my own history and life's lessons, sharing insights and understandings that I've learned along the way.

I've lived a full, colorful life filled with pain, drama and lots of lessons. Some are fifty dollar lessons, some are hundred dollar lessons, and some have cost a pound of flesh closest to the heart. The truth is, that pain is a great teacher and an impetus for personal growth.

I've had many mentors and counselors who've helped guide me through my darkest moments. They've lent me strength and support, without which, I would not have fared so well. Life has made me a little weird, but I like to think that it's my best feature.

Perhaps some of these stories will carry some enlightenment for you or someone you know and care about. Everyone in pain needs love, understanding, and support.

Do you know which herbs would be helpful when you're depressed? Do you consider getting a massage when your back hurts? Do you understand how a broken heart can kill you? These stories and more, will help guide you to consider the common sense remedies that our mothers may not have told us, or may not have even known about. The treatments are simple, but the effects, are profound.

The names and particulars, of the people in this book have been changed to protect their privacy.

Please tread water through the story of my becoming who I am, and skim through the science that is the backbone of the remedies suggested, make note of the suggestions for health and growth, and please, read on to the thought provoking stories, that have passed before my eyes.

This book is dedicated to *Love*,
in all its forms

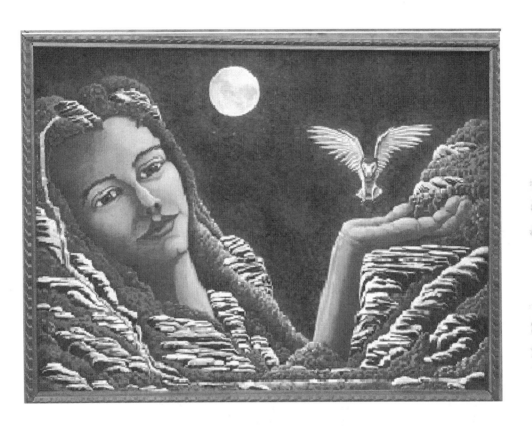

ALLOWANCE

*To allow knowledge and wisdom to alight
in the palm of your hand.
You must first
open your hand.*

—

Contents

Chapter 1
I am what I am.

An LSD experience when I was fourteen years old, revealed to me that I was sent to this planet to bring Love to the world. I remember waking up in the morning, at my girlfriend's house, looking in the mirror and seeing a huge temple, like the Eiffel tower. It was colored from top to bottom with the colors of the Chakras, one-half was filled with white light, and the other side was filled with black. I've seen this same type of temple since, in a book about spiritual enlightenment. But I saw it first, in my head, that morning, forty six years ago.

A truth once seen can never be unseen. Through mind altering experimentation, my life had nearly come to a spectacular and colorful end, all those years ago. The insights were precious and I had no intention of wasting the 'do over' that the universe had granted me. Why was I still alive? I knew it had to be for something important. I was left with the question, how do I proceed? What is my path and skill for bringing Love to the world? Where do I begin?

I'll begin here, by telling you that I was born in New York City. When I was very young, we moved over the Hudson River, and across the George Washington Bridge, into New Jersey. As a young woman, I drove a cab, back and forth across that bridge. I had the night shift and was terrified for my life. I decided to quit before I became a statistic, a young female, victim of violence.

My friends and I hung out like bums, down by the railroad tracks. They all drank and shot drugs, tempting death for a transient high. I had to call an ambulance, more than once. They hated me for saving their lives. They would rather have died, than have the cops come.

They stumbled around, looking like the living dead. I already felt like a freak, and I couldn't bear to look any worse, so for that reason alone, I never shot heroin or did coke. I may have drank too much, but I never lost my mind, or sold my soul, like they did.

I remember walking down to the tracks one evening, and seeing a pile of clothes laying in the lot. When I got closer I noticed it was shaking and shivering. It was Klinkie, a local junkie on the verge of death. I called the Emergency number, waited for them to get there, and left. I never looked back. I was done with that dark, dead end, chapter of my life.

One evening, traveling alone, on a midnight search for truth, I slammed my crappy little car, ninety miles an hour into a concrete bridge.

Not far from the accident, two young officers sitting in the local police station, could hear the crash from their desks. They both ran out to see what happened. I was apparently dead. The handsome young rookie called in a DOA, and holding no hope for my survival, stood there looking at the smoking wreck. After a moment of consideration, he pulled open the car door, and attempted to move the hair from my bloody forehead. Suddenly, and without warning, I took the opportunity to throw up all over his shoes.

Realizing his awful mistake, single handed, he pulled me from the jagged wreck and loaded my broken body into the back seat of the police car. I had smashed my skull, torso, arm and legs. Blood from my fractured skull was running down my face. My whole body was covered in fresh blood, and now, the entire back seat of the police car looked like a slaughter house. I drifted in and out of consciousness.

In the emergency room, I discovered that I was paralyzed down the right hand side of my body. Only half my face worked and only half my body could move.

After a few horrifically painful days in the hospital, unable to take pain killers because of my fractured skull, my skin started to peel off my body in sheets, like a lizard shedding its skin.

My spiritual vision, from so long ago, was vividly projected onto the inside of my eyelids. I was still alive! Once again, I knew that I had been spared for something important. Love and gratitude swelled in my chest.

My dad always told me, "Crying never does anyone any good, but laughing can get you through anything. If you can't laugh at yourself, kiddo, you're never gonna make it in this world."

I laughed at myself, well, half my body laughed, the other half laid there like a lump of clay. Working hard toward recovery, I welcomed the shock treatments, physical therapy, and psychological evaluations, as part of the healing process. I was disappointed that I couldn't drive until my brain stopped seizing.

I took my strength and solace from the 'me' that lives inside my head. I'd always known that there was someone else in there besides just me. So now, I relied on her more and more. I was determined to live, and ride the traveling zenith that was my life to come. Hand in hand, with the me inside me, I pulled a phoenix, and emerging from the ashes, I arose again, even stronger than before.

Many years later, after marrying the love of my life, I chose to follow the road less traveled. At the wizened age of thirty seven, I enrolled in chiropractic college. I was not just the oldest woman, but the oldest person in the program. Four years later, still the eldest, but now, the most highly honored student of the year, I graduated with a license to help and heal.

In celebration, I hired a rock and roll band, painted myself blue, and had a hippie party in the woods. I created an altar to myself, placing symbols of art and science, wisdom and lunacy, along with candles, skulls, and bones, atop of one of the biggest boulders I could find. Laughing and dancing with all my kooky friends, I phoenix-ed once again. My new name was Bluefish and I was reborn. I married myself and my profession. From the wreckage of my twisted dreams I became,

Dr. Bluefish,
At your service.

I was taught the scientific protocols to help people. But most importantly, I learned how to bring Love to the world. I learned that the best medicine comes from the heart, and I now had a way to share it.

I have a knowing that healing energy travels through the meridians of my body and emanates out through the palms of my hands. The energy of the universe is what heals, not people or things. In spite of all my education and training, love and understanding is the most important tool that I bring to the table.

Chiro is the Greek word for hand. The chiropractic profession is more that just cracking bones, It's working lovingly with the hands. To me, that means that true healing comes from the spirit, soul and energy matrix of the universe. All that universal Chi, flows from the palms of my hands.

We are all spiritual beings having the fantastical experience of a physical manifestation, in this world. Working with the physical body, affects the spiritual body, and vice versa. While working with people in this way, they have shared some amazing and bizarre stories with me. I share these astonishing true life stories, with you, in the coming chapters, attempting, through a curiously eccentric read, to impart wisdom as well as entertainment.

Every day I pray that I will be good at my job.

I work with the time, space, power grid, which to me, is the spaces between the molecules. I use love, wisecracks and jokes. I provide a place to laugh and a place to cry. Through mutual respect and heartfelt consideration we find guidance and wisdom for us both.

As a quick example, of an apparent mind body manifestation, let me tell you about a young woman who came into my office with a stiff neck. She was frightened and in pain, and couldn't turn her head. She needed comfort and understanding, Love, not drugs. She was already my patient, and she knew from experience that she would be safe and protected.

In talking with her, I discovered that this neck situation started when she answered the phone. She was feeling totally fine and happy until the phone rang, when she grabbed the phone, and she heard her mother's voice on the line, she had a physical reaction to her mothers voice. Her body froze, her neck twisted, kinked, and pain shot up into her head. She had to hang up the phone.

I knew this woman and it was pretty clear to me, and probably anyone else who hears this story, that it must have had something to do with the relationship that she was having with her mother. "Oh no, no, no" she said, "That's not it, I love my mother. It's definitely not that."

Now listen, I'm a mother, I have a mother, I love my mother, but I know that sometimes, we moms, are a pain in the neck!

For some of us, our mothers make us insane. We've all heard the Freudian belief that all of our emotional problems stem from our relationship with our mothers. I'd like to think that contrary to that world renown and universally accepted theory, not all my childrens' problems are my fault, but I know that sometimes, even my own nutty mother drives me crazy.

There are some people who believe that they've had a wonderful childhood and that their mother was a wonderful and sainted person. But, most of us moms are just normal people, and we make mistakes. Sometimes, these mistakes drive our children crazy. And, sometimes, once in a while, after a no good, very bad day, our children really don't want to talk to us, not even on the phone.

Life is like a spiral. When confronted with problems that we are unable to solve and reluctant to confront, we will continue to circle back to that same issue, over and over, often with increasing intensity. The situation may create a vortex of unreasonable and unremitting physical and emotional pain. This pain can seem unbearable, leading us to drugs, or surgery, or worse.

But honestly, drugs or surgery, usually don't work. These medical cures for emotional problems may relieve the pain temporarily, but the real problem or cause is still there, lying below the surface, lurking in the emotional swamp of unresolved, unrequited, and unwanted feelings. No matter what the cause, we must always consider love as part of the cure.

Extreme emotional anguish can be so overwhelming, that our subconscious mind attempts to save our life, by hiding the painful emotions in our physical body. This is the root of psychosomatic pain. It's important to remember that this psychosomatic pain is not fake pain. It's real pain. Emotions can kill you. When your heart aches, your muscles spasm, your joints twist, your nerves pinch, and your body really does physically hurt, a lot. Anguish can cause a heart attack.

The answer in this crazy mother, daughter, situation isn't pretending that there is no problem. The answer is in integrating, understanding and accepting the relationship, by working through the good, the bad, and the ugly, and not only tolerate, but find a place of loving kindness in our hearts, mitigating the effect it has on our lives. But, sometimes, the answer lies in realizing that your mother is toxic, and in that case, the solution may lie in creating boundaries that can save your life and your soul. But, ignoring the problem, that never works.

I recommended that this lovely, sensitive, young lady continue with chiropractic, mind-body care, and also incorporate psychotherapy into her life. Refusing to believe that her unresolved emotions could have anything to do with her neck pain, she ignored my advice and treated the episode as a physical unsolved mystery. Her neck pain became chronic. Massage, chiropractic, and sympathy helped but it was just a temporary solution to a big painful problem. Without confronting the hidden root cause of the situation, emotional turmoil would continue to lurk beneath the surface of her consciousness, causing physical pain and emotional grief.

After many episodes of her subconscious mind trying to get her to pay attention to the true mind-body pain connection, a more extreme condition manifested.

The last time I heard from her was after a Frisbee session in the park with her current boyfriend. She was planning a visit with her mom afterward. Somehow, during the game, she injured her neck, more severely than usual. She couldn't turn her head and she was crying in pain. She said it was like getting hit with a two by four.

Instead of visiting her mom with her new boyfriend, she visited the Emergency room. The doctor immediately recommended pain killers, muscle relaxers, and aggressively discouraged her from seeing a chiropractor, or anyone else who would massage or adjust her. She doesn't come to see me anymore. She's off from work, and has had several steroid injections in her neck.

Could it be that her mother was simply a big pain in the neck? Maybe that was why her subconscious mind decided to hide her childhood heartache and sorrow in her neck.

I'm not saying that every time you hurt yourself playing Frisbee, you really have a problem with your mom, but when there is a true emotional component involved with an injury or incidence, our emotions won't allow our bodies to heal. What starts out as emotional pain, over time, becomes an unrelenting true physical problem.

By the way, her neck continues to be a problem. The new boyfriend didn't work out, and now, instead of just severe neck pain, she seems to have stomach problems that just won't go away. It's nothing definite just a feeling of unease and discomfort. I wonder if that stomach ache gets worse when she is planning a visit to her mom.

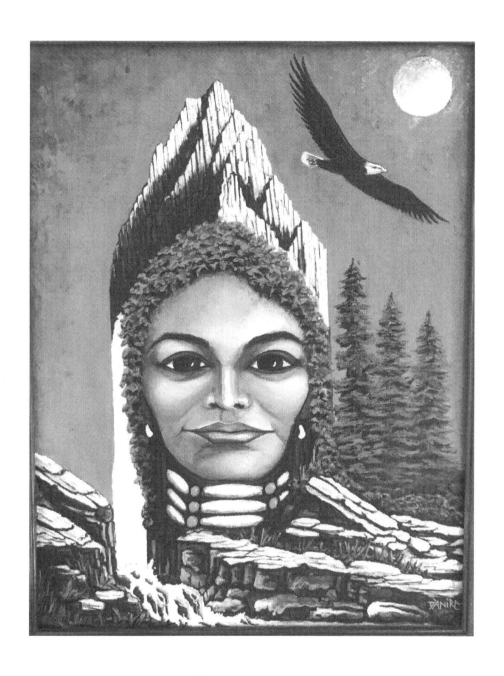

Emergence

breaking through self imposed boundaries,
to claim my personal power.

Chapter 2
Who's living inside of me?

I love to dance. It's one of the true joys of my life. Trudy threw a birthday bash with a band and a dance floor. We all showed up, dressed for fun, and we had a blast.

It's a small town so, everyone there was either a friend, or a patient, or both. Mostly both. That's the night that I met Claudine.

When Claudine walked into the room, everybody, male and female, turned their heads to look. Her strikingly beautiful long legs and silky blonde hair, were like tractor beams for eyeballs. She walked and dressed like a princess, even the cat was jealous.

Someone said, "This is Dr. D., She's an amazing healer." I hate it when people introduce me like that, I feel pretentious and embarrassed, even though, I'm not the one making such an exaggerated statement. Claudine gazed pleasantly and smiled at me benignly, not rude but not engaged. I was surprised when she called the next week for an appointment.

She came in complaining of chest, back, shoulder and stomach pain. I could see that she was trying very hard to hide her fear and pain. She was wound up tighter than a watch spring, (Remember when our watches all had watch springs?) I could tell by her presentation, that she really didn't want to be in my office, moreover, she really didn't want to ask me for help.

Initially, I felt more like her servant than her health care provider. I don't usually feel that way, but she had an air about her, exuding an aristocratic authority and command, that I knew better than to challenge, if I had any hope of helping her. She hated to admit that she had a problem, but the constant, severe pain she was experiencing, was frightening her, so there she was, at my door. I'm honored when people choose me to help them, reluctantly or otherwise.

Her power posture was a red flag, warning me to watch my step. She was used to being in control and in charge, and our relationship wouldn't work unless, I let her be the Boss. I could, of course, do my job, but I had to be very careful to gain her permission, before venturing too deep into her personal space. It felt like I was walking through a mine field.

She's was a tough gal to work with, but what Claudine had to teach me was unexpected and profound.

Claudine had never been to a chiropractor before, possibly because she didn't like being touched. I don't like to make blanket statements but, when a person reacts that way, it's usually because they've been hurt.

When I did start adjusting her, she said the sound of the adjustment frightened her. But, I bet the real problem was, that for the one split second it took to adjust her, she couldn't control the interaction. She hated losing control. Being in control meant that she was safe. If I couldn't get her to loosen up and trust me, helping her wasn't going to happen.

But it did happen.

Over time, she relaxed enough to let down her guard. Finally, she granted me permission to enter her highly protected, vulnerable, personal space. I started by massaging her neck, and piling hot packs onto her back. I stretched out her legs and, most important of all, for her, I listened. I never challenged or pushed her, that would have pissed her off and ruined everything. I just listened, and then I listened some more.

Through my chiropractic adjustments, I released some of the tension and physical mis-alignments that were blocking the flow of her Chi. When we finished, she always felt relaxed and relieved. She would leave happy, feeling better than she had when she came in. She returned fairly regularly with the same problems and with the same guarded need for help. Her aches and pains just wouldn't stay away. Our sessions helped her to feel better and get through the week. So, grateful for the relief, she always came back.

With each session, we talked on a deeper and more intimate level. I focused on the topics that she was obviously avoiding, because that's where the gold is. I heard the story of a bank robber, Willie Sutton, who, when asked why he robbed banks, said, "because that's where the gold is."   I ask painful questions, because that's where the gold is.

One evening, after a particularly deep adjustment, like a sudden cloud burst, Claudine, broke down into tears. "I miss Greg so much!" she blurted, "I wish he were here, I wish he was here! He was my only friend and he's gone. I miss him so much I could die. I think of him all the time. If only he were here, my life would be different. I don't know if I can go on without him!"

"Who's Greg Honey? What happened to him?" I asked.

"He's Dead. He's my baby brother and he's dead! He was sick, so very sick, for such a long time. I miss him so much and I love him so much. I love him more than I've ever loved anyone."

"You've been married twice," I said, "You loved him more than your husbands, more than your children?"

"I love him more than anything, or anyone I've ever known. I can't do this, I can't go on." She was crying the whole time and her nose was so stuffed up she could hardly breathe. I quietly handed her a tissue and let her go on.

She continued to talk about her little brother. It made her cry because she loved him so much. As children, they were each others' only solace. They clung to, and consoled each other, hiding from their parents and the world. They hid out in the closet under the stairs, not moving, trying not to make a noise, praying that no one would hear them in there, swing open the door to their private haven, and drag them out into the horribly real, loud frightening nightmare, that was their childhood home.

They promised each other that they would always stay together. But like Peter Pan and Wendy, Claudine grew up, got married, and left. Leaving behind, her delicate, baby brother, alone and unprotected.

Over the years, he became sicker and weaker, and was unable to move out, or move on. Eventually, his condition worsened to where he became hospitalized. The pains in his back, chest and stomach became so unbearable, that he stopped eating, not long after that, and not that long ago, he died.

That evening when she came to see me, after she burst into tears, she told me her story. We talked a lot about the crazy coincidence of how her pain started when her brother's condition worsened and became critical, and the further coincidence that the pains that she was now experiencing, seemed to be the exact same pains that her little brother was having, before he died. Once again, the tears slowly started running down her cheeks. Contemplating the connections, she began to cry some more.

That was when we both realized, she was keeping her little brother alive, by keeping him locked up inside her. Not allowing him to leave her, by carrying his sickness and his pain, lodged deep inside her own frightened body

I recently read a letter that Albert Einstein supposedly wrote to his daughter, Lieserl. He asked that it be held private until the world was ready for the truth. The truth being that when he proposed the theory of relativity, he forgot to include the force of Love in the equation.

Although the letter has since been labeled dubious in its authenticity, it very rightly purports that the missing force in his theory, was love. It states: "This force explains everything and gives meaning to life. This is the variable that we have ignored for too long, maybe because we are afraid of love, because it is the only energy in the universe that man has not learned to drive at will."

It was love, and losing the only person that she ever loved with all her heart and soul, that was the driving force behind Claudine's pain and suffering. I mentioned that if she wanted to get better, she had to let him go. Still crying she said that she couldn't, she couldn't bear to go on without him.

"Perhaps," I suggested, "we can find another way to keep Greg alive in your heart, another way to keep a piece of your beloved brother in your life, without your having to carry him around, through the pain in your body. Hold your love for him in your heart, but not the pain. Keep his memory, and the intense feeling that you have for him alive, by creating a sacred place to honor him in your life.

Create an altar.

Put the altar in a personal place that you see every day. Put his picture there and send him your love. Speak to his picture as though you are speaking to him.   Keeping your feelings locked up inside, is what's causing you all this pain.

Place pictures of the two of you together, some of his special things and loving mementos, write stories or poetry about him, and place all of it, everything, even the pain, there at the altar.

Honor his memory by sending him prayers of love.   Let it support you in times of need. It was love that was making her sick and it would be love that would cure her. In the end, it all comes down to *love*.

We can all do this when we are confronted with an emotional situation that we need to cherish, but not harbor as a burden. Make a sacred place in our homes to honor the treasured emotions or events of our lives. If it's painful, lay it down at your private shrine. Visit it later when you can make time to examine your feelings, cherish your memories, and be grateful for what you have.

Claudine had always insisted that her pain had nothing to do with her heart, she was thinking physically and I was thinking emotionally. She was so frightened to let go of his pain, that it would be like he was dying all over again, and this time, without his pain in her body, she would be abandoned and completely alone.

With two failed marriages, the longest intimate

relationship she had ever had, was with her little brother.

As we spoke, I adjusted her back, her neck, and everywhere that she was harboring her dead brother's pain, trying to loosen and release the emotions that had been locked up, deep inside.

Letting go is a process; it takes time and strength. When she left my office she was feeling so much better. There was a lightness to her that wasn't there before. She had a path, a plan, and the desire and determination to follow it through.

About a year after our work together, Claudine married a very handsome, and much younger, man. She seemed blissfully happy and it could be that this relationship will be a long lasting one. By releasing the crippling pain, she cleared some room in her heart for another man to enter, and he did. She could love her brother, and love her husband. Now, there was room in her life and her heart, for both.

Claudine taught me that we can carry truly incredible treasured moments and/or devastating tragedies deep inside our bodies. They can be cause for celebration or cause for pain and suffering.

I never expected a story like that to come out as a cause of back pain, but when it did, it made sense.

If you don't already have one, make a place in your home or your personal space, where you can keep your treasured memories. Taking the time to decide what items to place there is an important part of the process. Make time every day to visit and contemplate your sacred altar and the important feelings and emotions you associate with its contents.

Cherishing our pleasurable and painful memories, is both, healing and enlightening, and sometimes, life changing.

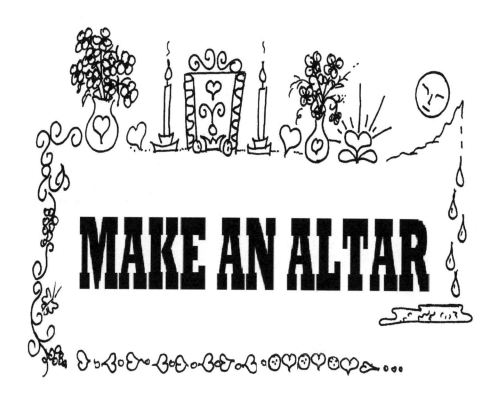

MAKE AN ALTAR

Chapter 3
Cereal Box Mensa

When I was young, I was a little peanut, tiny, sensitive, and quiet. Very very quiet. I learned it was better to be seen and not heard, and even safer, not to be seen at all. I learned how to watch and to listen.

I would see people doing things, and I would think to myself, "That's stupid. Why are they doing it that way?" When I ventured to voice my opinion, they treated me like I was stupid. Quite often, my opinion was dismissed, at first, because I was a girl, and then because I was a woman. I didn't look very smart, and because of the way I was treated, I didn't feel very smart.

They used to give IQ. tests in elementary school. I learned from those tests that my IQ. was around 160. I didn't know at the time, what that meant. But I knew that my dad was angry about it. My number was higher than my brothers, and he didn't like that at all. My dad was English and in our household, the boys were all that mattered. They inherited property, and they inherited the business, not the women, they did the housework, or just hung on the arm like eye candy.

When I graduated from high school, my dad gave me a choice, I could have a wedding, paid for by dear ol' dad, or I could go to college. I immediately chose college. He was shocked. Are you sure? He asked me several times. You won't have a wedding when the time comes.

Yes, I was sure, and no, I didn't care about a wedding.

But, even in college, when I ventured an opinion, the boys would smirk at, or ignore me. It was typical for women, at that time, to be overlooked, unless they were gorgeous, which I wasn't. The professors, however, would listen and acknowledge my thoughts. I was a straight A student, at the top of my class, when it came to science, biology or physics, I was usually right. When it came to doing things the easy way, I was always right.

When I graduated from university, Summa Cum Laude, I began to realize, that maybe, I wasn't so dumb. Fast forward to professional school and the graduate record exam. The GRE, which I took cold, ranked me at the top two percent of college graduates, in the world. Wow! It took that test to make me realize, after a lifetime of feeling inadequate, that I was actually intelligent. I joined Mensa, the high IQ society, and I found that, although I've always felt like a freak, I'm not a stupid one.

I cleverly display my Mensa certificate prominently on my office wall, hanging it, side by side, with my other diplomas and awards. Funny enough, even with all of my diplomas and honors, people are most impressed, and I'm sorry to admit, shockingly surprised, with the Mensa certificate. "Where did you get that!" one woman asked. "Cereal box." I replied.

I'm not so quiet anymore, but I am still sensitive, almost to a fault. I can feel when people are thinking about me. You know the feeling too, someone pops into your head and then – Boom – they call you on the phone, or you see them on the street and you think, "Hey! I was just thinking about you."

I thought of calling my practice,
"Psychic Chiropractic --
Don't call me, I'll call you."

Recently, I read some articles published on the Heartmath website discussing the studies done on the heart-mind connection and it's role in intuition. When a person is shown a series of beautiful or repulsive photos, in random order, the heart will react correctly to the *upcoming* photo, reacting even before the image is shown to them. The heart will beat calmly when a beautiful photo is going to be shown, and then, react wildly when an image of horror or gore is coming up next. The heart reacts, *before,* the image actually appears.

I have always thought that intuition comes from the heart, not the mind. These studies seem to confirm the precognitive qualities of the heart. I'm astonished to learn that this has been scientifically supported. These results have been duplicated more than once and by many different sources. I am further assured that treating people from my heart is the right road for me, and ultimately for my patients.

I work as a "lone wolf practitioner." I have no partners, and no employees. I'm the receptionist, the doctor, the cashier, the book keeper, the janitor, and the complaint department. My boss is tough, but she's fair.

My office is more than casual, it's a memento museum. I have so many treasures lying around, that I don't know where to begin. The balsa wood and tissue paper, model, biplane, hanging from my ceiling, represents a love affair between two artists. It was built by an academy award winning illustrator. He originally built the model plane for his, fashion designer, lover, and when they both died of too much wine and too little care, the cleaning crew threw everything out. No one remembered him when he died and I rescued the treasure from the dumpster, along with the monkey skull and Disney prints. It's frightening that such a remarkable and talented man could end up alone and forgotten, his treasures thrown in the trash. Not totally forgotten, however, I remember him.

The stuffed mallard and pheasant hanging on the wall, are payments, from a taxidermist with a bad back and no money. I have paintings, pottery, stuffed animals and hand made soap. All payments from grateful, but slightly threadbare clients. I have a sliding scale that goes down to zero, and I'm worth every penny. I work with warm hands and love.

I have found my way to bring love to the world.

Chapter 4
Vomiting up the past

"I've got this pain in my divorce, I mean, I've got this pain in my chest." As a Freudian slip, truer words were never spoken. She got that pain from her divorce. Roberta had gall bladder surgery to relieve the pain in her chest. Unfortunately, the surgeons couldn't remove the painful emotions that were causing the problem, so, they attempted to cure her, by cutting out her gall bladder..

Her story started long ago, when Skip was a young, strong, Kentucky, country boy, leader of the pack in the small backward town, where he and Roberta grew up. Roberta was an overachiever. Skip was not. Through the blindness of youthful desire, Roberta fell madly in love with the handsome rebel, got pregnant and got married.

After their first son, Sage, was born, Roberta, just as quickly, got pregnant again. Skip lost his job. Then their second son, Taylor, was born. Determined to keep the family together, Roberta went back to work and skip didn't. Through her determination and vigilance, the boys survived long enough to make it into kindergarten. Getting the boys into school, relieved Roberta of some of her worry. They were safer in school than they were with Skip, thank god for school.

As the days went by, Skip was doing less and less

and went missing more and more. He was worthless, but somehow always manged to have cigarettes and beer. By the time Skip went missing for good, it was a financial benefit to have him gone. Roberta was brokenhearted and relieved, at the same time. She tried filing for child support, but it didn't do her any good. Skip had skipped town and couldn't be found. Roberta shouldered the burden of raising the boys all by herself. That's when she first began to notice the small nagging pain in her shoulder.

She put up a good front, appearing fine and happy, while actually in deep pain. Like a bird, Roberta was remarkably good at disguising her pain and weakness, but the effort it took to maintain the facade, was exhausting.

Birds, like many wild animals, will attempt to appear healthy and strong, even when, in fact, they are horribly sick and weak. Weakness and vulnerability, in the wild, can lead to persecution and torture, or worse yet, death. In the bird world, the doves, the symbol of peace, are the worst offenders. In captivity, birds will, under stress, single out the weaker birds in the flock, and begin a campaign of relentless bullying, pecking at their backs, and ripping through the skin, until they finally succeed in knocking the weakened victims to the ground.

The strongest, most fit birds will then, peck off the dying birds legs, and end it all, by pecking the vital organs or the spine until the bird slowly and painfully expires.

The shocking truth about these beautiful, graceful, birds is that they don't kill quickly. They don't mercifully put the suffering bird out of it's misery. The birds at the top of the order, amuse themselves by prolonging the anguish of the victims on the bottom, pecking at their open wounds, never killing, but never allowing recovery. The result is an agonizing slow death. Survival of the fittest is a natural occurrence in nature, but torture, that surprised me. The life lesson in this case is; It's best to look good, even if you don't feel good.

Roberta was still a young, lovely, blonde, curvy, chic. She did her best to look good. You would never have guessed that she could hardly move her arm.

Years after Skip walked out on the family, her condition had become chronic and Roberta resigned herself to life long, intermittent shoulder pain. It all happened so gradually that she couldn't pinpoint the exact time that the pain began.

When the boys finally reached their teens, Robert found herself with a smidgeon of freedom and free time. She began meeting her friends at the pub for drinks and snacks. That's where she met Scott.

Blonde, blue eyed, honest, ethical, adventuresome, and strong in body and character, Scott embodied the virtues that every woman looks for in a man. After years of single parenthood, Roberta once again, fell in love. But this time, due to her history, she was suspicious of him and his intentions.

Her heart and her body, wanted Scott, but her brain

said, no. she wasn't willing to jump into a relationship, if there was any possibility that it might end up like the her marriage to Skip. She had followed her heart once before, and aside from her wonderful children, she still suffered from the episode.

Scott was so persuasive and seemingly perfect, that she opened the door to passionate sex, and her heart to a new love.

One pivotal day, test strip in her hand, Roberta walked out of the bathroom holding a positive pregnancy test, and she began clutching at her chest. Her life with Skip flashed before her eyes. Heartache, anger, and fear rose up to her throat. She had been romping around with Scott, for awhile, but it was all in fun and not serious. Her mistakes of the past were threatening to repeat themselves. She could not survive a similar challenge at her age. Thank goodness, the boys were in school, but what would she do with a baby!

Suffering from the still painful memory of her abandonment, Roberta was reluctant to take a chance on Scott. She learned from experience that trusting and depending on someone could lead to disaster.

After informing Scott of the situation, he pulled her to his chest and professed his undying love, affection, and loyalty, to her, the boys, and the baby, for the rest of their lives. Roberta struggled to resist his charming character, but she was so exhausted she was having trouble making decisions.

Time wore her down, Roberta chose to take the

leap. She would trust in love, and take a chance with Scott.

Her joyous relief didn't last long. Shortly after her reluctant decision to marry Scott, another surprise exploded on the scene. The other girl that Scott had been seeing, when he began dating Roberta, came by to say that she was pregnant, and the baby was Scotts'. Roberta sat there in silence and the other woman, let herself out.

When Scott found out Roberta was pregnant, he was thrilled and happy. He was ready to commit to her forever. When he found out he was having baby number two, with a girl he had stopped seeing months before, he was shocked and dismayed, and not happy at all.

Roberta's shoulder and chest pain became so debilitating that she went to a doctor who began prescribing anti-inflammatories and pain killers. The pain in her shoulder hurt less than the pain in her heart, and since she was uncomfortable taking the pills while pregnant, she used very few of them.

Despite the dilemma of two women and two babies, Scott was sure that Roberta was the love of his life and refused to let this other woman come between them. He agreed to provide financial support for his other child, but he loved Roberta and begged for her understanding and trust.

The shock of the unplanned pregnancy reminded her of Skip. Like being shot and stabbed, she clutched at the right side of her chest, and fell to the floor in tears and anguish.   How could she trust enough to love again?

Scott was relentless and she finally agreed to go through with the marriage. With all their friends gathered by the fountain in the park, and with Scott's friend, John, who got his minister's license over the internet, performing their ceremony, they became husband and wife. You could barely see the tiny baby bump, that Roberta was hiding under her billowy white dress.   All the women cried, and then we all had a big party.

As time went on, it became apparent that this other woman wasn't actually pregnant. She had just wanted Scott so badly, that she was willing to do anything to alienate Roberta and try to keep him for herself.

Six months after their wedding ceremony, Roberta, crying and screaming, gave birth to a beautiful, healthy, baby girl.   There was no mistaking that this, fair skinned, blonde haired, pink cheeked, bundle of adorable future trouble, was Scott's child. She looked exactly like him and was just as strong, healthy and loud!   Scott was in love and it's a good thing too, because when kids start growing up if we didn't love them as much as we do, we'd kill them.

Roberta's oldest son, Sage, grew up strong and handsome. After graduating high school he found work and a wife, in that order.

Taylor, unlike his older brother, was dark and gloomy. He ran with the bad boys looking for trouble. He hated school, his life, his home, the father who left him, and himself.   Trying to cope with his emotions led Taylor to drugs and alcohol. Like a runaway train, he ran the streets and then he stopped coming home.

Weeks passed with no word. Then, one day, after months of silence, the young man showed up at the house, sick and broken. Roberta and Scott stood beside him, refusing to give up on him. Taylor felt like an orphan and Scott wasn't his real dad.

Scott, a marine biologist, specialized in designing marine robots.   He made contraptions with arms, legs, levers and claws, that traveled deep into the ocean. Working on, or in the ocean, was his dream job and fulfilling his promise to provide for the family, he worked hard and was gone most of the time.   He traveled the country selling robots and training operators.

Roberta had one last test for Scott, could he stand by her and her incorrigible son, or would he bail out, abandoning her and her son, just like she always feared he would.

Scott loved Taylor just like the son he never had. The only solution he could think of was to keep the miserable, sullen young man by his side 24/7. He figured if he didn't let him out of his sight, he could catch him before he fell. Not everyone has the option to make "take your kid to work day," be every day, but Scott, with great sacrifice and fortitude, made it work. As a self employed entrepreneur, Scott began dragging Taylor around with him everywhere he went.

He tied Taylor to his side like a toddler to an apron string.

Nature is the best medicine for the soul, just sitting, for thirty minutes a week in nature can reduce heart disease, anxiety, depression, and improve health and vitality. We should all try going to the beach, the park, the hiking trails, or even just a place in the yard under a tree to sit and watch the birds. Being in nature can help everyone improve their emotional and physical well being, The body will also produce DHEA, an anti-aging hormone when we allow ourselves to sit in the healing environment of nature.

The ocean has healing qualities. Scott introduced Taylor to his new best friend, *the ocean*. He learned to dive and find his way around a boat. The spark of life was lit in his eyes and he fell in love with the sea and the creatures living in it.

Once a drug habit has taken hold, the connection can sometimes be impossible to break, but there's always hope. Roberta wholeheartedly trusted her son to Scott, and Scott proved his love for them both. Taylor today is finally free from drug and alcohol addiction. You might say that he is addicted to the ocean, the sun, and the sand. When he's not working, he's surfing.

Through it all Roberta's doctor prescribed gallbladder removal surgery, but that constant nagging pain never went away. The doctors had no other recourse and recommended she continue on anti-inflammatories and pain killers. Both of which, she used sparingly. Until she came into my office, she never considered that chiropractic could help solve the decades long,stabbing pain that had taken residence right between her shoulder blades. She had been living with this pain for so long that she didn't even mention it when she first came in.

The adrenal glands are small, triangular, little endocrine glands right over the top of the kidney. They are responsible for producing and balancing important steroid hormones essential for coping with daily life challenges. Aside from the sex hormones, estrogen and progesterone, the adrenal glands produce adrenaline, called the fight or flight hormone, and cortisol, the stress balancing hormone.

When the adrenals are constantly over-stimulated, like they were with Roberta, the adrenal gland itself becomes overburdened and fatigued, if something doesn't change, the next stage is exhaustion. The final stage is complete adrenal failure, and that's where the gland stops functioning sufficiently to maintain homeostasis. The glands failure to produce essential amounts of cortisol can lead to disease, mental breakdown, depression, irritability, insomnia and exhaustion.

Severe adrenal fatigue can also weakens the ligaments of the rib cage, allowing the long slender ribs to wobble and twist, which often results in causing a stabbing pain in the back. A twisted upper rib usually stabs right between the shoulder blades. Sometimes this chest pain can radiate down the arm, mimicking a heart attack, or a gall bladder attack. For the past fifteen years, Roberta had been treated for gall bladder pain that was actually caused by a twisted rib.

When she walked into my office looking strong and fit, I noticed that she wasn't moving the upper right quadrant of her body. I gently moved her to the table and we began to talk. I talked to her body through my fingers and her body spoke back, through a subtle language all its own. It's not a fixed protocol, it just happens when you start to touch people. Behind her lovely mask, she was hiding pain right behind her heart and at the level of the gallbladder. Those organs are the house and home of love, fear, bitterness, and anger.

After heating and massaging her, I adjusted her neck, her thoracic spine and low back. Last, but certainly not least, I adjusted her rib on the middle, right side of her chest, right at the spot where her gallbladder had been before the doctors removed it. Boom! It was a loud impressive movement. She immediately yelled out, "OH GOD! Wide eyed with surprise she screamed at me, "My pain is gone. My gallbladder pain is gone! I had surgery to remove that pain, but it never went away, but that did it! What you just did took the pain away!"

After the seeming miraculous adjustment, she right away started talking about Skip. When people have a huge body release, the first thing that comes into their heads is the hidden cause that they usually never talk about. I have found through the years, that twisted ribs usually have names on them. The name on Roberta's rib was Skip.

She was so grateful for the relief, that she was totally open to making the lifestyle changes that would allow her body to heal.

To nourish and repair her crashed adrenal glands, I started her on a product that is made from adrenal glands, called a glandular, for non-vegetarians, it's the best place to start. For vegetarians, an herbal formula of Licorice root, Withania and or Ginseng, is equally effective, along with daily vitamins and minerals.

I also recommend a short daily stretching or Yoga routine for everybody to help repair and relax our stressed out bodies.

Roberta had been drinking coffee all day long to kick start and keep her going throughout her day. The caffeine wasn't doing her exhausted body and adrenal glands any favors. I know from personal experience, that caffeine can be highly addictive and Roberta drew the line at eliminating coffee.

After starting her on a regime of vitamins, minerals, essential fatty acids, adrenal supports, meditation, yoga and journaling, she voluntarily cut down her coffee intake to one or two cups in the morning, still a lot of coffee, but better than a pot or two a day. All things in moderation.

With the new lifestyle changes, Roberta was a new woman, but that rib was still a pain and she would occasionally visit my office for relief. Life had given her a second chance at love, but the ghost of her first love still haunted her life.

Scott had more than proven his love for Roberta and the family. Love flourished between them. With the kids finally grown and on their own, Roberta gave in to Scotts' desire for outrageous adventure.

Scott signed them up a for a healing excursion deep in the mountains of Peru. It was an adventure with a purpose. Everyone on the trip was there to heal some painful unresolved emotional trauma. Roberta and Scott hiked deep into the forest and took part in a hallucinogen induced, healing ceremony. After swallowing the magic potion, the group of seekers were led to a healing waterfall located on the side of the mountain. The water was beautifully clear, streaming in rivulets, and shimmering down the rocks.

Gazing at the gorgeous waterfall at 13,000 ft., she began to feel severe anxiety and pain. Her emotions and her stomach were swirling. Fearful of a heart attack in the jungles of Peru, her life flashed before her eyes. Leaning against a rock, she vomited. Heaving, retching, and clutching for dear life to the sides of the rock, she had an epiphany.

She vomited up Skip. That's what she said - she vomited up Skip. Her anxiety vanished. A weight was lifted. Her chest opened up for the first time in decades. She was free from the pain, anger and bitterness that had been restricting her life and vitality. The next part of the journey was spent in a cave with the guide playing the Pan flute.

When she spoke to me afterward, she said that she was finally free from Skip and the bitterness and anger that was undermining her health and her ability to be blissfully happy. The love in her heart radiated like the sun. She experienced a miracle, an emotional exorcism, and feels like a whole new person.

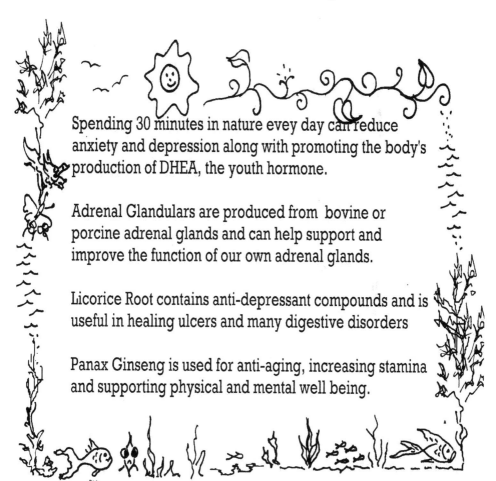

Spending 30 minutes in nature evey day can reduce anxiety and depression along with promoting the body's production of DHEA, the youth hormone.

Adrenal Glandulars are produced from bovine or porcine adrenal glands and can help support and improve the function of our own adrenal glands.

Licorice Root contains anti-depressant compounds and is useful in healing ulcers and many digestive disorders

Panax Ginseng is used for anti-aging, increasing stamina and supporting physical and mental well being.

Chapter 5
The Mashed Potato Mountain

I've made my home and office in a small town in Southern California. The population is eight thousand, fruits, nuts, weirdos, winos and aliens. There are so many people riding the razor's edge between genius and lunacy, that the whole town vibrates with eccentricity. We are an open minded, forward thinking bunch, and all of us, out of the box.

I like to think that I was drawn to this place, just like in the movie, "Close Encounters of the Third Kind." In that movie, Richard Dreyfuss was so obsessed with a vision in his head, yearning for a place he'd never seen, that just trying to sketch it out or describe it, wasn't enough. One night at dinner he stole all the mashed potatoes and started to sculpt his geographical vision out of the mashed potatoes. That's how it was for me, I was destined and determined to find this place and live here.

Growing up between Queens, New York, and Fort Lee, New Jersey, was like an initiation by fire. As soon as I could walk, I began to run away. After graduating from the university, I finally found someone who was willing to run with me. We had no destination, we were running from, not to. So, along with the love of my life, I drove in our converted school bus from the East coast of New Jersey, to the West coast of Oregon. We drove until we hit the ocean and we couldn't drive anymore, driving our 'house on wheels' right up to the rocky edge of the Pacific Ocean.

Aside from getting the heck out of New Jersey, the other half of my heart's desire was to get married and have children, so, when we finally parked the bus at Seal Rock, we took the leap.

Leaving our hugely pregnant, Yellow Lab, and wily, little black cat, locked up inside the school bus, *home alone*, we checked in with the county clerk to be married. Holding hands, in hippie rags, we waited in line at the courthouse. With two total strangers, agreeing to be our witnesses, the anonymous clerk, pronounced us, husband and wife. After our official kiss, we ran off, hand in hand, through the crisp, clean, Oregon air. With joy in our hearts, we looked forward to a future filled with love, laughter, and adventure.

Swinging open the metal door that led up to the drivers seat of our rolling home, we were stopped dead in our tracks. Squirming around, between the gas and brake pedals, were eight of the cutest little yellow, puppy meatballs, you've ever seen. The new mom was resting under the dashboard, feeding her babies. None of us was going anywhere soon.

I loved living in the green forests of Oregon, but it didn't love me. I became pregnant and was joyously, anticipating the birth of our first, beautiful baby, but soon after I got the good news, I miscarried, losing my precious treasure.

I was heartbroken, but determined to try again. In pretty short order, I got a second chance, but after a couple months, I lost that little baby too. I was stunned, shocked, and alone in my grief. One more time, I thought, third times a charm. But not this time. No charm for me.

This last time, I carried my baby into the second trimester, and this miscarriage was much more dramatic. I remember sitting on the toilet, doubled over in excruciating anguish, my hair and my tears hitting the floor. The pain in my gut was nothing, compared to the pain searing through my heart. The child I had always dreamed of, the child that I was going to love more than anyone had ever loved me, was slipping away.

My husband didn't mind the idea of having a baby, and as it turned out, he is the best father I have ever known. But, back then during our hippie days, it wasn't his dream to have a kid and he didn't share my grief, nor understand my heartbreaking trauma. I felt like my chest was cut open, and my heart was ripped out. I was having a near death experience, and he was having a beer.

Beyond broken, I couldn't stay there, in that place, any longer. My grief, depression, loneliness, and unhappy memories were overwhelming. We packed up our stuff and started driving on down the road.

With our compass pointing toward the sun, we gave up on our Oregon dream, and began our California dream. We settled in a small town in the mountains about 100 miles from Los Angeles, called Luna. The Air is clear, the people are friendly, and the undercurrent is rebellious non-conformity. I knew immediately that we were home. I had found my mashed potato mountain.

Like a rabbit, I once again became pregnant, this time, in southern California. I dreaded the possibility of losing another baby, but I wanted a child so badly that even though I was frightened, I was willing to take the chance. Month after month crept by. I passed the critical period and held onto that precious little tadpole, longer than ever before. Day by day, I prayed that maybe, this time, my miracle would happen.

One afternoon, sitting in front of the TV, with my hand lying across my pregnant belly, I chanced upon on a documentary based on the area in Oregon where I had been living when I had lost all my babies. There were a bunch of mothers talking about how all the mothers in that area, during the time that I had been living there, lost their babies in the early months of pregnancy.

It seems that the government had been spraying defoliants to nurture the pine trees and support the lumber industry. The defoliants caused miscarriages to everyone who came in contact with them. I remembered that while I was living there, trucks would come by and spray something all over the place. One time, they even sprayed me.

No one was taking any responsibility but the

producers were reporting on the situation. The women in the area had petitioned to have the spraying halted. Their ardent protests and the facts of the documented health concerns won the case. They stopped spraying the poison. The result was that everyone, who had been miscarrying their babies, began to have full term healthy babies.

It was a miracle that I had turned onto that station at that moment. I mourned my losses, but rejoiced that maybe, just maybe, it wasn't me. It wasn't that I was unable to have children, I was just in the wrong place at the wrong time. I had hope.

My due date came and my baby didn't. Everyday was a torment. Not just because I was as big as a house, but because I was frightened that something was wrong. What if it wasn't the defoliants, what if it was me. Maybe there was something wrong with me and mother nature knew that I shouldn't have any babies.

Two weeks past the due date, after hours of labor, I finally gave birth to the most lovely little girl I've ever seen. My heart broke open and I discovered a kind of love that I've never known before. I now have three children, whom I love more than life itself. I thank god for them every day.

I was never happy in my childhood home and I always wanted a happy home of my own. Once my first little girl was born, I wanted a safe place for us. A home that I would never leave, and that would always be there, for all of us, forever.

I made Christmas ornaments on my kitchen table and sold them to Leaning Tree Corporation. I hid away every penny in a coffee can under the sink. After selling the school bus, we finally had enough money to make a down payment on a tiny house with a big yard. Our Shangri-la was originally a pig shack. But I was thrilled to have it. When you start with a hovel, the only way is up.

The are two types of weather in Luna, drought and flood. During our first big storm, I fell asleep to the sound of raindrops on the roof. In the middle of the night, while we slept in our bed, the rain came down in buckets. In the morning, when I plopped my feet down onto the floor, I splashed into water up to my ankles. Turns out, my silly little house was built in the flood zone and we were, wall to wall, flooded.

My Husband and I decided to fix it ourselves. We ran telephone poles right through the middle of the house, from one side to the other, then we put house jacks under the whole thing and inch by inch, we lifted it out of the mud.

That was thirty five years ago, and I'm still here in my pig shack. When I first started my chiropractic practice, my friends, my family, my ex-lovers, and even my sweet ex-husband, all got together and built me an office out of the garage.

Jeanie, Suzie, Christy, and the rest of my female warrior friends helped me build the walls, hang the drywall, and paint the floor. When Dennis, a barefoot, mountain man, ex-boyfriend, came to do the drywall mudding, he said "It looks like a bunch of women put this place together!" And we did.

Even my friend, the local shaman, Joseph Four Bears, and his Lakota wife came to bless the space, wearing beaver tails and carrying an abalone shell, they burned sage and brushed away the bad Juju with an eagle feather.

My converted garage may not be pretty, but it's mine, and I love it. The whole place, kind of looks like Pee Wee's playhouse, if Pee Wee was a Luna, California, wild woman chiropractor.

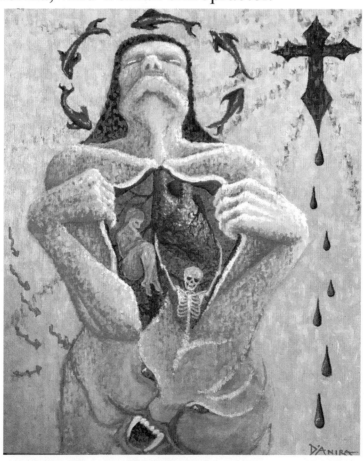

Chapter 6
I can't get up

One of the sweetest people who has ever bounced into my office, is a Blonde, mop top, mother of two, wife of one, hardworking, lovely woman named Zoey. She is one of my favorite patients, who exudes openhearted happiness with a warm honest smile and rosy cheeks.

My favorite 'Zoey story' is the one where she found a tiny bird lying in her yard. It had flown into her window and looked like it had broken it's delicate little neck, and died. Overwhelmed with motherly emotions, she reverently picked up the lifeless body, and cradled the still warm creature, gently in her loving hands. Wrapping herself and the bird up in her blanket, she sat, resting against the back wall of her house, and called up her BFF, to share her grief.

Bundled in her blanket, she sat petting the silky feathered, lifeless bird, while she tearfully shared her feelings with her best buddy on the phone. Grieving and praying under the California sun, she jumped in astonishment. The confused little creature had opened its eyes and resting safe in her hands, sat there blinking in the sun. Filled with Joy, Zoey nuzzled the little beak. When she was done celebrating the miracle, she stood up to release the fluffy feathered angel back out into morning sky.

That's Zoey, – she loves everybody, -- her kids, her husband, her friends, all, just like she loved that tiny bird.

I have an antique phone on my office wall. It's a wooden box with a bakelite speaker and a crank on the side. Most kids don't know what a rotary dial phone is, even less an antique relic, like mine. Zoey's young daughter, Lark, loved playing on that phone while I worked on her mother. Chattering and chirping, pretending to be my receptionist, she spoke haughtily, to imaginary customers, making them appointments, and scribbling make believe information on my new patient intake forms. It was totally adorable, and in her young mind, she was the boss.

Zoey's equally amazing, intelligent, handsome son, Cliff, decided as a young teenager, that he was going to be a buff body builder. He didn't just began to work out at the gym, he began studying nutrition and the bio-mechanics of weight training. He lifted weights, but he wisely balanced his strength training with stretching. He took supplements regularly and ate organic, non-gmo foods. He worked slow and steady, retaining his hardy good nature, and at the age of eighteen, he was buff, fit, kind and wise.

What more could a mom want, right?

Cliff and Lark graduated from high school and were both leaving home. Cliff for South America, where he would explore the wilds of Costa Rica. And Lark was headed for Europe, where she and a girlfriend, would carouse around Europe living *la vida loca*.   They had both been accepted into prestigious colleges and were looking forward to college life. But first, they were going to take a gap year, anxiously looking forward to seeing a bit of the world. I often think that I need a gap year. Maybe, we all do.

Coincidentally, my daughter, before she started her career, went off to school in Costa Rica, leaving me beside myself with worry and grief. The address where she was staying was something like "The pink house at the end of the street with the crooked palm." How can that be an address?

One day, when she had been gone for several weeks, she called me and excitedly boasted, "Guess what I did, Mom! Don't get upset, I'm calling you because I already did it, and I'm still alive." "What! What! What did you do!", I practically screamed into the phone, anxious to hear what crazy, dangerous, nonsense, she had gotten herself into.

"All my friends were going to see the bullfights but I didn't have enough money to go. They said if you sign up to fight the bulls you can get in for free. So I fought the bulls!"...... *my breath caught in my lungs*. I didn't drop the phone, but I wasn't able to speak, so she continued. "Diane took pictures, so you can see them on Facebook. All day long they've been beeping their horns and screaming "Torera! Torera!" I guess that means lady bullfighter. The local TV has been playing it all day. I'm famous! They gave me a shocking pink cape to match my hair! Pretty cool, huh?"

Well, no, I didn't think it was pretty cool. For the moment, I was seriously distressed. The fact that she did something like that at all, left me traumatized. What would she do next? I could beg her to be careful, but I have been doing that all her life and it obviously wasn't working. By the way, I didn't tell Zoey that story, not yet, not until all her babies were back safe in the country.

Lark and Cliff had been planning their trips for months and Zoey had been getting, increasingly, more anxious. Her panic and fears were escalating, and her visits had becoming more and more frequent. Even Lark, came in more than usual, stressing over her impending international adventure.

Zoey came in for nebulous, non-specific low back pain. The low back is the base of the chakra system, and energetically, it's the seat of the soul, and associated with family and finances. It seemed obvious to me, that in Zoey's mind, her family was disappearing. Her children were, for the first time, leaving home, leaving town, and leaving the country.

As mothers, we want our children to grow up and become responsible adults, but when they go, we grieve horribly over their absence.

"Are you taking your withania?" I asked. Withania, also called ashwaganda, is an adaptogenic herb helpful in balancing mood swings and in giving the body a positive boost. It's also a general tonic to our system, helping the body deal with, and adapt to, different levels of tension, anxiety and depression. It is sometimes useful for sleep disorders and fibromyalgia, among other things. She said, "No, I've run out. But, I should probably get some more because it really does seem to help. But lately, nothing seems to help. I just don't know whats wrong with me."

That was the perfect opening for me to tell her a story from a similar situation in my life. As opposed to the bullfighting story, which was sure to increase her unease, I shared the feelings of pain and emptiness that I went through when each of my three children left home. My daughter left for Hollywood, my oldest son joined the Air Force and I was especially bereft when my youngest son, my last little bird, left for New York.

I became too tired to go out. I felt so weak and exhausted, that I couldn't get out of bed. I didn't know what was wrong with me. I decided that I was getting old and I just needed to rest. I decided that the best thing to do would be to lay in bed as much as possible, and only get up when I had to go to work. Once at work, I felt better and happier. But, when work was over and the day was done, alone with myself, I was tired again. Not just tired but, exhausted. *Maybe I have Cancer, I thought. Maybe I'm dying!* I felt like crying, and I didn't feel like doing anything.

I was depressed. I was heartbroken. But, actually, I was experiencing the '*empty nest syndrome*'.

Any parent, or caregiver, can get it, man or woman. All parents are happy to have their children grow into adults and leave the nest. We're proud to see them start their exciting new life as an adults. Some of us turn the child's old room into an office, or a crafting space.

But for some of us, it's devastating. We're not the least bit happy to see them go. We have spent most of our adult lives, loving, hugging and doting over our little angels. We've built a huge part of our lives around them, hovering and helicoptering, so they don't die. We've prayed over their sleeping heads for their health, success, and longevity. Hurting when they hurt, and jumping for joy when they succeed.

Having said all that, now that we have raised them to be self sufficient, courageous, and intelligent young adults, we must sit back and watch them walk off into the big world on their own. It's scary, it's painful, and it's almost unbearable.

When I realized the truth of my condition, I forced myself out of bed, and, once again, I began to take my supplements and my herbal remedies. I exercised and went to work. Just recognizing that I was in a state of depression, didn't make it go away, but it's a start. I forced myself to work and to walk. Every evening I walked briskly around the block.

The best way to pull yourself out of depression is to exercise. The chemicals of emotion that are produced by the mid brain when we are depressed, fill our bodies with sadness. When we just sit around, the chemicals build up and are metabolized too slowly to be completely eliminated. When we continue to be unhappy, the chemicals build up, layer upon layer, until we become so overwhelmed, we are unable to move our legs. To metabolize these hormones, reducing their effect, we must get up and move.

One of the easiest things to do is to get up, and walk, for at least twenty minutes. Every day is a good start but, twice a day would be better.

Even when you don't feel like it, **get up and move!**

I also recommend taking a withania herbal formula, along with your daily vitamins, minerals, and essential fatty acids. Essential fatty acids, contained in fish oil, flax seed oil, and walnut oil can be especially helpful in combating anxiety and depression.

As a general, all around tonic, I recommend echinacea. Yes, I take it every day, and no, it's not bad for you to take it every day. It actually improves your overall health, vitality, and cognition. When using herbs and vitamins, please, choose wisely, you get what you pay for. The inexpensive brands are not usually the best. I recommend, whole food organic supplements and organically grown herbs.

Thank goodness, Zoey has friends. She has people who can see what's going on and call on her to go out, to walk, to talk, and to share her feelings. We all need people with which we can share our feelings. For some of us, it is our spouses, our friends, or even our pets.

Having a job to go to, got me up and out. I felt better, once I realized, that what I was feeling was normal, for a woman who had cared for her children, for twenty five years, and suddenly they were all gone. No, not literally gone, but gone from my apron strings, gone from my arms, and gone from their beds, and from the rooms that they had lived in all their lives.

Over the years, my children have blossomed and grown, started young families of their own, and now know the difficulties of parenting. I am so proud of them all. I love them with all my heart and I love the grandchildren that they have blessed me with.

Zoey continued to be a hot mess. I was too, when it had happened to me. It takes time to move through the challenges of life.

Lark and Cliff went off on their foreign adventures. They were learning new things, but they were so young. For us parents, who are left behind, getting back to work, whether around the house or in outside employment, is a huge help.

The herb I recommend to combat depression is withania, or ashwaganda, adding a little ginko biloba wouldn't hurt either. Some people respond better to st. john's wort. If one remedy, is not working, try another. Personally, withania and echinacea work for me. That's what Zoey used, along with the stress relief of exercise, the healing effect of sharing her feelings with friends, and, last but not least, finding a purpose in work or play. Following those recommendations can help break the unhappy, downward cycle that we *empty nesters*, can fall into.

As far as our beloved babies are concerned, we can only hope and pray for the best, answer the phone at any hour, and go on living our lives with purpose and love.

We hold our children like tiny birds in our hands, and when they are ready, we release them out into the universe, like angels in the sky.

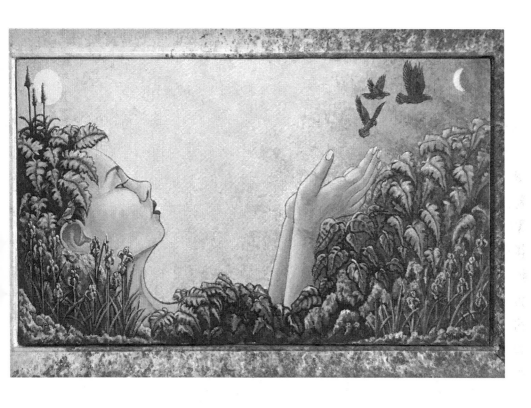

RELEASE

Releasing my precious treasures
out into the universe.
The sun is rising behind me.
The moon and the mysterious future lie ahead.

Chapter 7
Bitterness, the party pooper.

Of all the ways to kill yourself, bitterness is the most cruel. It's the invisible psychic killer that strangles joy and happiness, leaving angry bile in it's wake.

I have a friend who is dying of bitterness. He's always been so cynical and haughty. So wrapped up in his own self importance and pain, that he refuses to see that his stubbornness and pride are his own worst enemies. His once courtly manner has morphed into anti-social irritability. He clings to his anger like a lover, pushing away anyone who challenges his attachment. He won't forgive and he can't forget. Forgiving is gracious. Every day he is less and less gracious. His emotional irritation may have created his irritable bowel syndrome. He blames his sour stomach on his disease, instead of seeing that his anger, resentment, and accusations of others, can cause the very symptoms that are making him sick to his stomach, causing such horrible pain.

The world is full of bloated people. Their indigestion and intestinal inflammation are symptoms of the way that they look at the world. They come to me because they are in pain. It's impossible to tell, just by looking, if the pain is from a physical trauma or an emotional one. But, once they start talking and explaining, I can usually tell the difference.

These people hold their pain, grief, sorrow, and

resentment locked up inside their bodies. These unresolved feelings can morph into an emotional situation, that irritates their nervous system, effects their digestion, and alters their behavior. They lock themselves away, afraid to share, afraid to let go, afraid that without their pain, they will have nothing.

In order to heal, we must be willing to release our anger, and embrace forgiveness. That's why friends and relationships are so important. Friends help us see the humor in our hardships, and the hope in our future.

Life is hard, but it's harder without friends. One of the hardest, but most important things to do in life, is to find a friend and be a friend. Friends are mirrors to our souls. They help us to look at ourselves, help us to grow, help us to heal, and help us to see the importance of forgiveness.

Friendships boost our immune system, lower our blood pressure, and help us handle the stresses of everyday life. They make us healthier in every way. I recently read a study investigating the most important factors for longevity. The single most important activity that a person can do to increase their life expectancy is to hang out and socialize. Friends and lovers help us to live longer.

Our bodies release a friendship hormone called oxytocin, sometimes referred to as the gather and nest hormone. It's produced in both men and women. During an attack, men gather and prepare to fight. Women, on the other hand, during intense times of stress, produce large amounts of oxytocin, which leads them to gather with their children or other women, huddling and nesting, protecting and nurturing themselves, and their families

Oxytocin is also the bonding hormone in both sexes. Oxytocin levels are elevated after orgasm, for both men and women, leaving everyone in a blissful and endorphin fueled state. Levels are especially high in women who have recently given birth and are breastfeeding. It permeates the young mothers' body with feelings of comfort and contentment.

Even men succumb to the siren call of oxytocin, producing in all people, the need to bond and couple, and possibly fall in love. We all follow the pied piper of oxytocin. Friendship can satisfy a need that oxytocin creates, with or without love in our lives, friendship supplies a primal need for socialization.

Friendship, like marriage, is work. Nurturing a friendship takes time and consideration. Taking the time to connect and be there when they need us, as we hope they will be there for us. I'm not talking about the thousand and one friends on Facebook, I'm talking about a friend who really knows you. One who meets us for coffee or events. One who remembers our struggles and our accomplishments and who talks with us, laughs with us, and sometimes, cries with us.

I have a dinner party every week. I invite my special friends, and sometimes, I invite those friends that just need to be included for their own good. I always invite that grumpy, depressed, angry friend of mine, that I mentioned in the beginning of this chapter. The camaraderie helps us all to get through the week, and through the tough spots in our lives.

I recently attended a seminar on a condition called SIBO, which stands for, small intestine bacteria overgrowth Yes, I know, every week there is a new disorder that becomes the dubious problem of the month. This condition makes sense to me. The problem starts when the the bacteria in our gut gets out of balance. When the bad bacteria overwhelms the good bacteria, we get bloated, and have indigestion. The serotonin that is normally produced in our gut, is no longer produced as abundantly as it should be. Serotonin helps us to be happy, so obviously, lower levels of serotonin, makes us less happy. Our stomach, and intestinal imbalance, can actually make us grumpy, or grumpier, depending on the individual.

The recommended remedy for the situation involves first, clearing the gut with herbs of myrrh and artemisinin. Myrrh---that's the stuff that the three wise-men, were said to have brought to the baby Jesus as a treasured offering.   After the cleanse, we then reintroduce good bacteria to insure the proper procreation of the good stuff. My grumpy friend and I agreed to try the protocol together.

After several weeks, I can tell you that I feel great! My friend seems happier as well, although he doesn't like to admit it. He's not ready for that. But, I'm his friend and I can tell a difference. Friends are also good for noticing changes in our behavior, because sometimes we are too close to see them for ourselves.

Deep friendships are said to increase our endorphin production, thus, increasing our overall feelings of contentment and bliss. Having friends is one of the few things we can do that will naturally fight off the feelings of depression and anxiety. Wow! That sounds worth the effort.

If connecting one on one is hard, join a group or a club, go to the same coffee shop every day, sit for a few minutes, work on your computer, read a book or knit. There are groups in every community and they are usually posted in the local news or city website. Look for common interests and continue the effort. Practice by just showing up and keep showing up.

If you already have a friend, call them. Maybe put down this book and call them right now. Laugh about this silly book you're reading that reminded you of how much they mean to you. An endorphin release is just a phone call away.

Roberta didn't choose to be bitter. She moved away from her home and community when she got pregnant. That's a time when women need friends and family the most. She bravely chose to grab life by the tail, and it was often overwhelming. Thank goodness she is strong and tough, or she and the boys wouldn't have made it. When Skip deserted them, she had no one to talk with, or confide in, during one of the most difficult and confusing times of her life.

A wise counselor would be a blessing at times like these. If you don't know one personally, hire one. It's worth it, in the long run.

Roberta was open to friends, and when the time was right, she was still open to a relationship, even after Skip. Not every one can travel to Peru to contact our higher realms and release our bitterness and anger, but not everyone needs that. Friends, lovers, family, priests, counselors, groups can all help guide us to the same end, spiritual vomiting, instead of physical vomiting.

It's interesting to note that bitterness along with anger, depression and melancholy, can all be created and exacerbated by an irritated stomach, gut and digestive organs. It's not just that being depressed can effect your gut, but your gut can actually cause depression.

The gut has neurologically active cells similar to your brain. Serotonin is one of the major neurotransmitters in your brain. Your gut has been shown to produce the exact same chemical. Serotonin release can cause a feeling of happiness and well-being. The balance of good and bad bacteria in our guts directly influences our moods. Possibly by effecting the release of serotonin and other neuropeptides, by the nervous cells, in the gut lining.

Once again, life is about balance. Balancing the many strains of good and bad bacteria in our body, influences our digestion, our systemic pH, and the release of serotonin. Nerve impulses travel along cranial nerve ten, the Vagus nerve. This autonomic nerve carries communications from our gut, directly to our brain. The gut and the brain are friends--they talk all the time.

To help overcome the painful and deadly feelings of bitterness and depression, try taking nutritional supplements of prebiotics and probiotics, along with the difficult task of eliminating sugar and saturated fatty acids. Perhaps try the cleanse and replenish protocol that I have included at the end of this chapter.

One last thing about keeping friends and lovers that I learned from Supreme Court Justice, Ruth Bader Ginsburg, is her secret to a long and happy relationship. When she argues with a friend or loved one, and horrible words are said in anger, she pretends to be deaf. She drops the words from her mind. She just did not hear them. For that moment in time, she became deaf. It's the perfect exercise in self preservation, you just say to yourself, "I didn't hear that", and completely erase it from your mind. Don't look back, don't try to evaluate its intensity --you just didn't hear it-- you're deaf to it. Done.

SIBO cleanse

The best way to start to cleanse your gut is to eliminate sugar from your diet.

The cleansing protocol that my grumpy friend and I used, was this:

Myrrh and Artmisinin for four or five days, four times a day.

Then we introduced the good bacteria into our gut by taking tablets of probiotics for the next week.

We then repeated the cycle.

We could have used fermented foods along with kefir, or yoghurt with active cultures, but tablets were easier for my friend.

Chapter 8
I'll be home for Christmas

Bear with me through the indigestible description of digestion to assimilate the concept of the assimilation. *Remember, there will be a quiz at the end of the chapter.* Just Kidding!

Heartbroken and stressed out, Yolanda was exhausted, overweight and in pain. Her irritated skin, bloated belly, and tired eyes, betrayed her outward mask of strength, fortitude, and well-being. Beneath the layers of makeup, she looked sick.

Four months ago, her husband left her for another man. She was devastated, confused, and in pain. She tried to to be understanding and compassionate, but she couldn't pull it off. She radiated anger like a bonfire. What she really wanted to do was punch him, kick him, strangle him, and make him pay for all the years he lied to her. He selfishly stole her youth and innocence, under false pretenses.

Assuming the warrior stance, and using her body as a crock pot, she put a lid on her pain, and slow cooked her unhealthy emotions until the toxic stew began to make her sick.

Her kids and her friends seemed to have more sympathy for Don than for her. The feelings among her friends were, "He's the persecuted one," saying, "Poor man, after years of hiding who he really is and suffering for so long, at least now he can be himself." They sympathized with the "poor unhappy soul, just trying to find his way." "And besides," they thought, "How could she have not known?"

He had always been a kind and caring husband to Yolanda, but now that he had made his choice, he deserted her completely. After finding happiness and love, he turned his back on his former life and wife, and moved forward into a new world. He adored his children and included them in his *new* life, inviting them to meet his *new* friends, and live in his *new* house, in his *new* neighborhood. Everybody was welcome, except for Yolanda. He didn't want her there. Probably because she was so angry at him. All her loved ones were at his new house having fun, enjoying his new life, but not her. Naturally, she felt alone and betrayed.

She had always thought how lucky she was to have found such a sweet understanding man. He even liked to go shopping. Thinking back, he always had better taste in clothes, in décor, and in everything. Without Don, Yolanda was set back seventeen years. She had no idea that he was gay, how was she supposed to pick another partner without the fear of picking another gay one?

Yolanda dressed in black like a mourning shroud. She was so shocked and heartbroken that she withdrew into her house and spoke to almost no one. Some of her friends tried to call, but she wouldn't answer.

So, they all rallied around Don. They were celebrating and partying because Don was still out there, in more ways than one, dressing well and socializing. Yolanda wasn't.

For Don, his life was just beginning. His life with Yolanda, except for the children, was joyously forgotten.

Without an outlet for her emotions, Yolanda's life was a sudden nightmare. After the shock wore off, she was left broken and broke. From a partnership, to a left in the dust, half the bills became all the bills, and Yolanda spent every night alone with a bottle of wine.

The children loved being with their dad and couldn't understand why their mother wasn't happy for him. He was always the fun one anyway. Annoyed at her depression and resentment, they ignored her need for support, and avoided her texts and calls.

She knew she needed help, but her traditional doctor only offered her drugs. She didn't want drugs, she wanted advice and support. Her truly concerned friends, recommended that she see their wonderful, kooky chiropractor.

Dragging herself into my office, she presented with a myriad of aches, pains, and problems. Finding remedies for maladies is a puzzle I enjoy. Yolanda wasn't much of a puzzle, she was depressed, confused, and dazed. All of her symptoms, headaches, bloating, fatigue, depression, along with neck, shoulder and chest pain, believe it or not, could all be brought on by *stress*.

Her history and examination revealed system failure in many areas. Her digestion, the most important system for the assimilation of nutrients, was blocked by a stomach tied in knots.. Instead of digesting her food, it was rotting, and fermenting in her gut, producing gas, bloating, heartburn, constipation and sluggishness.

Through muscle testing and organ reflex points, I discovered that her stomach wasn't producing the all-important hydrochloric acid, and her pancreas wasn't producing enzymes. Working together, acid and enzymes break down proteins, carbohydrates and fats.

One of the first organs to be effected in times of extreme stress is the stomach.

Without HCL and enzymes, you can't have proper digestion and you look like Yolanda, a hot mess. Along with her digestive woes, her spine was misaligned in so many places that her body ached all over. We chiropractors call these kinks and pinches, *subluxations* or *mis-alignments*.

Our bodies, are electromagnetic generators and have circuits that must remain free flowing for our nervous system, and all other systems of our body, to function. When these circuits become blocked, our electrical circuits and Chi, which control every movement and function in our body, can't properly flow and we end up with sickness or disease. Chiropractic adjustments can open up these blockages and help relieve the problem.

I began addressing her issues one step at a time. After the first adjustment, she broke down into tears on the table. The adjustments released huge amounts of locked up tension and sadness that she was trying to keep hidden inside her body. Breaking into sobs, she began to admit how angry, hurt, and devastated she was with her husband, her children and a lot of people whom she thought were her friends.

She'd been hit by an emotional locomotive. In her

new picture of life, she had no one to turn to and no one who cared. All her life she'd been alone. She was a lonely child, so she didn't notice that although she had been married for thirteen years, she'd been alone the whole time. This apparent nervous breakdown was a long time coming.

As a weekend dad, Don and the children had all the fun. As a weekday mom, she was handling all the challenges keeping the kids clean and healthy, getting their homework done, getting them to school, and last but not least, keeping them out of trouble.

It's the same stuff that she always did, but before now, she had Don as her partner, and he helped with money, appreciation, support, and, of course, with fashion advice.

My holistic treatments for Yolanda included physical adjustments, nutritional supplements, lifestyle recommendations, and emotional support.

Now comes the part where you bear with me through the indigestible description of digestion to assimilate the concept of assimilation.

All the grief and tension were effecting her digestive system, and she was unable to properly digest her food. The first, and most important remedies that I gave her, were tablets of hydrochloric acid (HCL) and powdered nutritional enzymes. These two supplements are the place to begin when there is indigestion. They are easy to get at the local health food store. I told her that these tablets must be taken every time she eats in order to reduce her gas and bloating and increase assimilation of her food and heal her gut.

Step one: Skeletal adjustments. Step two: Digestion support. Step Three: Psychological counseling. Moving forward I recommended psychological therapy, which she said she couldn't afford. After some discussion, we agreed that keeping a journal and finding a woman's group would work for now. She desperately needed some friendly support. Looking through the local newspaper we found several groups that could be helpful to her. she felt better already. Love, support, and chiropractic care can work wonders on your soul.

On her next visit, she reported feeling so much better. Her stomach pains had dissipated and the bloating and flatulence had disappeared. She had connected well with the people in her woman's group and that alone offered her relief through shared emotions and experiences.

Her ongoing emotional cyclone not only effected her digestion, but also her hormones. Yolanda's constant state of nervousness, fear, and turmoil was causing her body to remain in a constant fight or flight mode. This condition is common in the jungle where animals are in constant fear of being eaten, but the body isn't made to remain in this heightened state of stress for very long. Reacting to her high anxiety, her adrenal glands were overproducing adrenaline and cortisol, which was pushing her adrenal glands to the point of exhaustion, and Yolanda, to the brink of collapse.

Normal levels of cortisol are necessary for proper body function. Under chronic stress our cortisol levels get out of control which can cause dangerous health problems involving our thyroid, blood pressure, immune system, bone density and muscle tone. Visually, cortisol deposits fat on our belly. We can't lose belly fat because our cortisol levels are too high. This belly fat can be the underlying cause for deadly disease such as a heart attack or stroke. Clear proof that our emotions can kill us.

In order to address this deadly situation, I prescribed an herbal remedy of Licorice root and Rehmania, along with an Adrenal glandular, all of which are available in the health store or online. A fifteen minute yoga regime would provide gentle stretching and promote relaxation. Her previous adjustments helped her to feel tons better. After each adjustment her body became stronger and more settled into a proper alignment. She didn't get this messed up in one day and it was going to take a while for her to recover. She was on the right road.

Yolanda found a new friend, Becky, in the woman's group and they met during the week for walks around the neighborhood. Her new friend provided support for her feelings. Becky wasn't Don's friend, so she could give Yolanda the unconditional support that she needed. She could freely vent her true emotions. Having a friend, like Becky, is as important as food.

Exercise, talking, and laughing provide the best cure for anything. By commiserating with Yolanda, Becky helped Yolanda to release her pent up anger. Getting those feelings out into the open, allowed Yolanda to move forward into a new life of her own.

Resting more and actually sleeping at night was a difficult, but necessary, task. Yolanda was being kept up at night by the thoughts spinning in her head. Using an herbal calmative of: Valerian root, Passion Flower and Hops, along with relaxing meditation apps., that we found on her phone, helped her to sleep. I told her to close the bedroom curtains, extinguishing any light source in her room, to help her stay asleep, once she got there.

It really is true that time heals all wounds. After several months on treatment, Yolanda began to feel a lot better. She still missed the life and the love that she once thought she had, but her feelings of betrayal and anger were diminishing. She was starting to enjoy her new friends, and she loved her new job. Progress like that doesn't come easy. Yolanda worked hard for it.

On her first Christmas after the breakup, she was preparing for a lonely holiday. Her kids made it clear that they preferred celebrating at their dad's house. They told her they'd see her later on Christmas day for their presents.

Christmas Eve used to be her favorite time, but now, it was the hardest. She still set up the tree and played her favorite version of "The Christmas Carol", but as the evening fell, her heartache was unbearable. She sat alone on the couch, letting the tears roll down her cheeks.

Looking out the window to the street, she saw her teenage daughter, Camille, pull up in front of the house. With joy bursting through her sorrow, she saw her three children pop out of the car with presents in their hands.

Pulling open the door with the tracks of her tears still streaking her face, she clutched her beloved children to her chest in a huge hug. Overflowing with love, and laughing with joy, they told her,

"It's just not Christmas without you mom!"

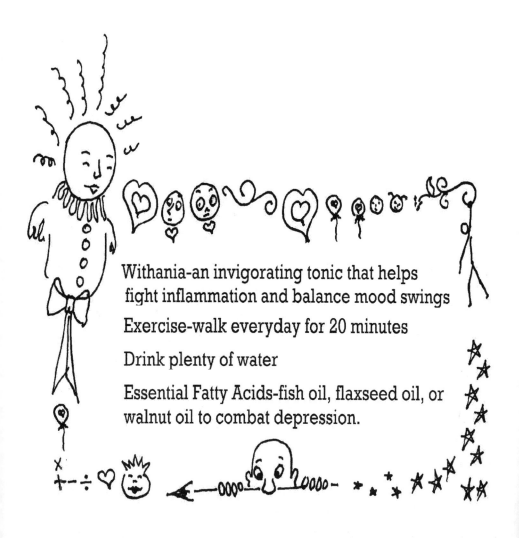

Withania-an invigorating tonic that helps fight inflammation and balance mood swings

Exercise-walk everyday for 20 minutes

Drink plenty of water

Essential Fatty Acids-fish oil, flaxseed oil, or walnut oil to combat depression.

Chapter 9
I forgot about that

The human body is basically a skin covered bag of electromagnetic chemical reactions. Our daily interactions cause peptides, neuropeptides and hormones to be created and released and ultimately, carried to every cell in our bodies. These molecular messengers effect our emotional, physical, biochemical and spiritual state, and essentially, every and all the reactions of life that take place within us.

Dr. Candace Pert, PHD., became Chief of Brain Biochemistry at the National Institute of Mental Health (NIMH) in 1983. She is one of my heroes, and should have received a Nobel Prize. Dr. Pert called the chemical messengers in our bodies, 'molecules of emotion'. She explains this and many other interesting biochemical reactions clearly in her book, "Molecules of Emotion." She was a major early proponent of mind body medicine and she believed that our daily experiences cause the release of molecules called neuropeptides which are produced by neuronal cells. These neuropeptides cause the manifestations of emotions, along with all the other biochemical reactions, necessary for our physical existence.

Other chemicals of emotion, called hormones, are produced by the endocrine glands. The difference in terms has to do with the cells that produce them. The effects of the chemicals are felt throughout our bodies and they create and affect all of our feelings, emotions, physical manifestations and bodily functions.

For example, stressful situations alert the adrenal glands to produce the hormone Adrenaline, thus creating a fight or flight sympathetic response.

These molecules of emotion are used to regulate body function, resulting in positive and negative bio-electrical-chemical reactions. They communicate with all of our organs, muscles, glands, nerves, and brain cells, to create feelings of hunger, thirst, love, hate, and every physical and emotional manifestation that we know.

In this hectic age, we hardly have time to completely relax, before the next emergency or alarm is sounded. The previously released stress biochemistry is never completely metabolized and eliminated, hence it builds up from one event to the next. The body matrix that never relaxes, stores layer upon layer of stress related molecules, until the viable ratio is exceeded and a psychological breakdown occurs .

Muscle spasms and knots are common areas where these chemicals of emotion are trapped. With massage and chiropractic manipulation, the trapped chemicals and waste products can be released from these physical prisons and proper function can be restored.

All of our mental and physical activities are

channeled through the electromagnetic pathways in our bodies, called the energy matrix. This electromagnetic, oscillating web, guides our conscious and subconscious, actions and reactions, creating the symphony we call life. By using this web, we can, like the internet with the cloud, communicate and interact with the innate intelligence of our being.

In my practice, I use a form of muscle testing that works with the emotional link between muscle pathways and the energy matrix. These pathways work like a gateway to connect our subconscious mind to our physical body.

To work with this muscle testing technique, I find a strong muscle and then I ask the patient a pertinent question. I challenge the muscle's strength immediately, pushing quickly against the force of the muscle. If the muscle stays strong against resistance, the question is considered unimportant or negative. If the muscle weakens after a question is asked, I the question is important, or positive.

I rarely use this muscular emotional response technique, but occasionally, I am so baffled with a patients lack of progress, that I open my chiropractic bag of tricks, and pull out my emotional response testing.

Elizabeth reluctantly ventured into my office one day. At forty three years old, she was tall, tanned, and toned. She looked like a gorgeous female Tarzan. She was a personal trainer in an exclusive health spa for years until she finally broke free and realized a life long dream of opening her own gym. She was proud to be running her own business and was very successful at leading classes in Pilates, spinning, yoga, and weight training. She had to be fit in order to lead her groups, showing, by example, how life's hurdles could be overcome. She expanded her programs and wisely turned her business into a corporation. She was an 'in charge' woman and enjoyed being her own boss.

She married Jeff, when they were young, and the two of them left Kansas together, moving to California where they could start fresh. Elizabeth liked being in charge and she made the decisions and most of the money, for both of them. Everything went along just fine, until her business went through a tough time and she needed Jeff to help and make some money. He tried to explain that he just couldn't find a job, no matter how hard he tried. No one would hire him and he was exhausted from the effort.

She realized then, that he was a bum, and that she had allowed him to be one. She didn't realize that they had made an unspoken contract, she did everything and he let her. With the struggle she was having now, the arrangement wasn't working anymore, and she began to resent it. She demanded that he do something. After that, she noticed he wasn't around much. He started seeing other women. He was looking for fun, and Elizabeth wasn't fun anymore.

The marriage ended with him stealing what he couldn't destroy, and driving away in one of their cars. His parting shot was to scream at her as he slammed the door, " You're a cold hearted bitch Elizabeth!"

After the debacle of a marriage to Jeff, her trust button was broken. Actually it was probably already broken before she chose Jeff. She dated men who worked a little, but never seemed to get anywhere. They usually moved in with her and she'd end up paying for most of their living expenses. With each of these live-in situations, she would eventually realize that she was being used, and a huge fight would ensue. The result was the worthless guy leaving in a storm of anger and accusation.

The Jeff scenario played over and over again. Each new man would scream at her and call her a bitch. But, that was after they took her for everything they could get. She wanted a strong loving relationship, but she didn't know how to find one or how to be in one. She was the only person that she could rely on.

She came to me because the pain in her neck and shoulders was almost unbearable. Her image was that of a powerful female body builder. Her neck pain was threatening to topple her empire and destroy her life. She tried many different healing techniques and as many different healers, searching for something or someone to relieve her pain and restore her mobility, but, so far, nothing had worked. At this time, she was unable to handle any of the challenging classes that she had designed for her groups. Without help she was headed for disaster.

She was in terrible physical pain, but also obvious emotional turmoil and extreme anxiety. Treating her like a porcelain doll, I had to use gentle, non-force techniques to get her to relax.

On top of everything, she was certain that the last therapist shouldn't have pulled and yanked on her neck like he did, she was certain that it was worse after his treatment, but she refused to confront him.

We worked together using massage, trigger point therapy, ultrasound, heat, and stretching. Slowly, she began to feel some relief. She felt much better and more hopeful after each of our sessions, but the improvements didn't last. Thankfully, she could at least get through her work day. It was frustrating for both of us.

She couldn't strong arm her way through life anymore. She needed to get some rest, and allow herself to heal. She was going to have to restructure her business. She needed to find someone to trust, and allow them to take over some of the work and responsibilities.

She began to see a new man. The good news was this guy was different from the rest. The bad news was, this guy was different from the rest. She was uncomfortable with change. This guy was perfect for her, but could she handle a mature responsible partner? Not being in charge was frightening. Between trusting someone to help her at work, and trusting this new powerful man, her neck pain was unbearable.

Acting out of exasperation with our push me-pull you success routine, I suggested we try talking to her subconscious mind through her body's energy matrix. I explained a little about emotional response muscle testing, and all the voodoo like interactions that it entailed. She was so desperate, she'd try anything. I took a deep breath, and after centering myself, we started. I asked her to lie on her back, raise her left arm, and make a fist. Explaining the procedure I said, "I'm going to ask you a question and then push on your arm. I want you to resist the push and keep your arm straight."

I thought about the main categories that influence our lives. They're the same for everyone--finances or work life, our childhood family or family of origin, our adult or current family life, and our love life or lack of it. If I asked a question and the arm stayed strong, then the question was irrelevant, if the muscle went weak and her arm moved back, it meant we hit gold, or the answer was yes.

"So, why is your neck hurting you, Elizabeth?" "Is this about finances?" The muscle went weak, meaning, yes. "Is this about family?" The muscle went weak, yes, again. "Is this about your love life?" The muscle stayed strong, the answer being no. So, it's about family and finances. " Is it about the family that you have now?" Answer, no. "Your family of childhood origin?" The answer, yes. So you see how it goes, every question has to be worded for a yes or no answer. Yes to finances when she was young. So, now I'm wondering how young. I break up her life into tens and ask about each decade. Was it in your 40's, your 30's, 20's, 10 years, 9, 8, 7. Yes! Seven years old is a yes.

How do I reconcile this information? Her present condition was from financial difficulty that she had when she was seven years old. It didn't make any sense to me.

"Elizabeth, your body is telling me that your condition is a result of a financial situation that you had when you were seven years old. I know that sounds ridiculous, but that's what I get. It also seems that it's not just your finances, but also involves your childhood family." Financial problems when you were seven, I knew I must have made a mistake. But, to my surprise, Elizabeth started to cry, small sobs slipping out at first, and then uncontrollable, deep sobbing.

With tears running down her cheeks, and snot out her nose, she told me a story of when she was seven years old. It seems that her parents had been struggling in southern California. Her parents were always fighting and her father wasn't working.

One day, after a long and loud bout, her father had dropped her, her mother, and her baby sister, off at a bus station. He drove off in a cloud of dust. They waited on the curb, but he never came back. They had no money, no food, no hope, and nowhere to go. Her mother was confused, and deserted, rubbing at her neck, she sat crying into a handkerchief. Instinctively, Elizabeth started rubbing her mothers shoulders, and telling her that everything was going to be alright. They sat like that all day, until finally her mother starting begging for change.

Soon after, the three of them crammed themselves into a tiny phone booth. She and her sister were squeezed in between their mother and the cold, glass walls. Elizabeth was just tall enough to be able to hear the conversation. She listened while her mother dialed her parents. Embarrassed, frightened and terribly, terribly, hungry, she listened as her mother cried and begged for help, pleading for money to buy bus tickets and come home. Home to grandma and grandpa's house, somewhere in Kansas.

She heard the desperation in her mother's voice, and the hard tone of her grandparents on the other end of the line. She was terrified for her mother, her baby sister, and for herself.

Our core beliefs and coping mechanisms are formed before we are seven. That type of emotional terrorism traumatizes and affects a person forever.

She decided right then, at the tender young age of seven, that, like Scarlet O'Hara, she would never go hungry again. She would never be at the mercy of some man, and that, someday, she would have enough money to take care of them all. Her grandparents, reluctantly and with great sacrifice on their part, were able to send them the money they needed and they went home to grandma's house.

She told me that she had forgotten all about that. "How could you possibly forget that?", I thought. But, once again the mind is an amazing organ and it can hide painful thoughts and memories, in order to protect us from ourselves.

Could all of her current pain be a result of the fear and abandonment that she had suffered as a child? Was it difficult for her to trust men because her father had proved untrustworthy? Had she been choosing losers for lovers because her father was such a loser? Could she change her life and her destiny by overcoming her fears?

When her mother was faced with ruin, she began to rub her neck. Did Elizabeth's neck pain begin when her financial worries began? The more she worried, the worse it got. The worse it got, the more she worried.

While she cried and retold the story, we worked together to move the fear out of her body and subconscious mind. By bringing those old memories into the light and into her consciousness, she would be able to examine and manage the fear and pain. Perhaps, her muscle spasms and neck pain were the result of years of piling everything onto her own younger shoulders. The fear and anguish she was feeling at seven years old was, all these years later, still locked up inside of her, and now, the adult Elizabeth was strong enough to confront the shocking, painful truth.

Maybe she needed to forgive her father. Maybe she needed to forgive her mother. And maybe, she needed to forgive herself. But, the anguish and bitterness was eating away at her soul. Opening Pandora's box of childhood trauma, helped to clear the burden, and shine a light on the shadows of childhood trauma and financial ruin.

After the miraculous results of the muscle testing technique, her condition began to improve. I adjusted her body while she consciously tried to let go of the past, and release the pent up feelings from her youth. She found a good counselor and therapist and shared her story and fears. She was, finally, able to work longer and with less pain.

She courageously moved her romantic relationship to the next level and became a fiancé. She had never before, truly allowed anyone to share her life or her financial burden. She also, let go of the fierce control she had over her fitness corporation. She took on a partner and let them become involved in the design and execution of the progressive classes that she offered.

Her childhood abandonment had left her unable to trust. Seeing the emotional roots of her situation helped her to overcome some of her protective mechanisms, relaxing her boundaries enough to allow true love to enter.

After her wedding, she sold her business, and moved a little further up the coast. Her new husband had an incredibly lovely ocean view ranch near Santa

Barbara.   I think that she said it was near Ronald Reagan's old place.   She had never felt better and I haven't seen her since.

About a year after our work together, I received a package in the mail. When I opened it up, there was a bright red scarf and a card inside. Elizabeth had personally crocheted this scarf for me. The card said that she was very, very happy and that she and her new husband were looking forward to their incredibly promising future together. She wrote that she was very grateful for our time together and thanked me with all her heart for working so lovingly with her. I keep the scarf in my office as a memento of her gratitude, and a reminder that childhood memories can haunt our lives forever.

I learned just how incredible the mind body connection can be and that it can actually be accessed through gentle emotional response testing.

Whatever the deep truth of the problem is, find someone to talk to about it, muscle test about it, write about it, release it, drink plenty of water, stretch, take a deep breath, exercise, and let it go!

Forgiveness is the key to moving forward.

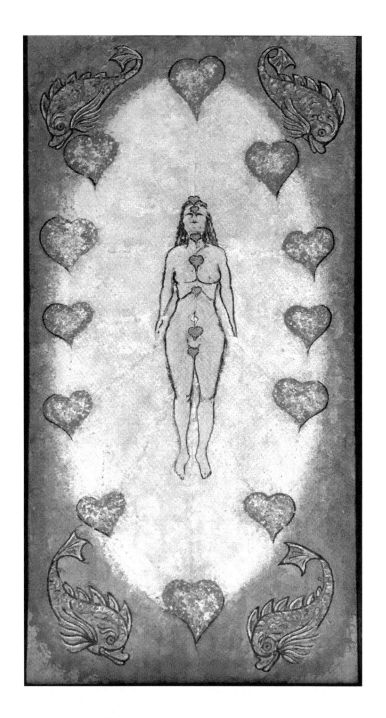

The energy matrix

Chapter 10
The freak in the grotto

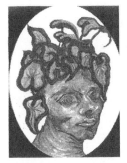 So When I first saw this place, where I live now with my three lovely children, all I saw was home. This half acre, where the playset stands, used to be filled with pigs. This house, that has become our home, was a pig shack. Over the years, it has moved from hovel to house, and from house to home. I plan to stay here for my forever, taken out, dead or demented, whichever comes first.

I was standing out in the front yard one morning, watching my little, two year old play in the dirt with the dog, when I heard this amazing laughter fill the air. Until that day, I was devoid of friends. I had my kids and my husband, of course, but a woman without girlfriends, is a sad woman, indeed. Friends make our walk through this world less isolated and girlfriends make a tough hike enjoyable! Walking out into the street, in search of the laugh-ee, I found Suzie. Suzie, the new neighbor, was sitting in her yard across the street watching her three year old play in the dirt. We became fabulous friends at first site. Now, Suzie has been my best friend for twenty-eight years.

Her son and my son are inseparable. Time or distance means nothing to them. I would say they were blood brothers, but these two surfer boys have ocean water running through their veins. From the salt water of the womb to the salt of the sea, they've been in the ocean since before they were born. Our two sons, and Suzie and I, are joined at the heart, and our families are joined by joy, laughter, and love.

Over the years, Suzie and I have weathered many a storm. Her marriage fell apart at the same time as mine did. Our mutual life trauma brought us even closer. Our families supported each other during devastation and celebration. No matter the need, we'll be there for each other.

After her divorce, Suzie had a series of short worthless relationships, before she met and fell in love with Christy. I wasn't sure how I was going to fit into this new situation, but I knew it would work out. If Suzie had a new best friend, I could be her sister. Whatever happened she was like blood to me.

The bisexual thing was surprising to me, but Suzie said she was in love with a woman before she married her husband, and now she was in love with a woman again, no big thing.

Christy was intense. Just her gaze was unsettling. She was a true artist. Her paintings were the reflections of her tortured soul, with graphic scenes of lust and love, colorful and disturbing. Suzie brought one of Christy's paintings home to hang in her house, a multi-colored female nude with huge vibrant wings flying over a deep crevasse, a strong, muscular arm was reaching out from the deep chasm and attempting to grab the winged woman by her delicate foot. Christy painted her fears in clear metaphors.

By day, Christy was an interior designer, faux painter. She magically transformed the walls of the wealthy, from southern California drab to warm, vintage Tuscany. At night, like many anguished artists, she would drink, way too much, and paint, way too late. Too little sleep and too much drink doesn't stabilize an unstable person, not an uncommon scenario among high IQ individuals. Christy was highly intelligent and also, just a bit, bipolar. But, a 'bit' is all it takes. She was highly functioning when she was on her meds.

People of both sexes were attracted to Christy, and I could see why. First of all, she was all the things I wasn't--handsome, tall, and lanky with lovely, long, dark, shiny hair. When she wasn't riding her motorcycle with her hair safely tied up, she allowed her satiny dark tresses to cascade beautifully down her slender back. She dressed up in tough black biker clothes, leather boots and tight jeans.

My favorite outfit was a cream colored poet blouse worn with her black leather vest. I envied her style, but I, being quite short, sadly had no hope of pulling off that look. I knew from experience that I would look like a mushroom in an outfit like that.

To supplement her sporadic painting gigs, Christy worked in an animal hospital. It was easier for her to relate and get close to the little, suffering and frightened animals, than it was for her to get close to people, it's a common trait among abused or neglected children.

With people, she kept her distance. Her cool, tough, reserved personal style, and a wise-cracking, "jokes on you" personality gave her an aloof quality that she was comfortable with. She was smart, sharp, beautiful and certifiably nuts. Like many psychiatric patients that I've known, Christy didn't like taking her meds. I've had some friends who attempted suicide when they stopped taking their pills.

It didn't take long for Christy to move in with Suzie. My friend, Suzie, had moved from across the street, to a house at the top of the hill and her new house was way cool. She rented the place from a local actor and actress, who for health reasons needed a warmer climate. The house was more than unusual, it had a strange personality. The piano was left behind by the previous owners, and I would play it when I visited. The piano seemed haunted, of course, I have no evidence, but when I sat down to play, I could feel someone else's energy playing along with me.

Ever since Christy entered the scene, whenever I went over to visit Suzie, I'd run into scores of interesting and unusual gay women. Suzie's house was the new hang out. Before Christy, I always found an opportunity to visit my friend, after

Christy, It seemed harder to find the time.

I worked out of my home, mainly so I could keep an eye on my kids, but also because it saved money, I didn't have to pay for office space or child care. When I first started my practice, I interned in an office downtown, but when one day I came home to find the house full of kids and the place beyond a mess. I knew I had to make some changes and be more present. Besides, now, when I have time between patients, I can wash the dishes.

When all the action started happening at Suzie's house, the kids started disappearing over there a lot. The atmosphere was way more party-like at Suzie's house and they liked it there. I didn't blame them. I thought it was a lot more fun over there too. There was always something unusual and fascinating going on at her house. I didn't have much time to hang out. My time and energy was exhausted making money and keeping my kids healthy. The school projects were the worst, we always seemed to be hitting up against the deadline date. The darn kids always waited till the last minute to tell me they desperately needed poster board or sugar cubes. I wanted to hang out with the gang at Suzie's, but I was too tired or too busy. I longed for the old days when we all hung together and made school projects, like kinetic egg carriers, or Egyptian pyramids. Christy didn't do school projects.

One day, a trailer appeared in Suzie's driveway and it became the home for Joanie, a desperately struggling, but proud construction working dyke. Suzie was loving and helpful. Letting Joanie live in the driveway was her way of helping.

At night, at Suzie's, when the kids were asleep, the hot tub under the stars and beneath the limbs of the old, twisted, oak, became the place to drink wine and smoke pot.

I was happy for Suzie, but I deeply missed the close friendship and support that we used to share.

Christy made me feel uncomfortable. She was cool, funny and hip and constantly poking fun at me with a "just kidding" cover. But, and it was pretty obvious, she wasn't kidding. Looking back I think she was suspicious and uncertain of my relationship with Suzie. I liked her anyway, I couldn't help it. If I was going to continue my friendship with Suzie, I was going to have to put up with Christy.

Among other things, Christy suffered from chronic neck pain and headaches. Out of compassion, our mutual friends, pointed her in my direction. She called my office, saying "Hey, I hear you're a bone cracking, miracle worker. I need a miracle, can you find some time for me?" Well, of course, I could, that's what I do. I figured, she could be tweaked from either painting walls all day, cranking and craning her neck, or from all the personal drama and trauma that she'd experienced in her life. Her personal life, I was to learn, held just as much cranking and craning as her professional life.

Examining and palpating her neck and shoulders, I could tell immediately that, first, she didn't like to be touched and, second, her muscles were like granite. She had obviously been carrying a lifetime of tension in her neck and shoulders. Judging by her defensiveness and muscle tone, her life must had been like 'Mr. Toad's Wild Ride'. When I massaged her shoulders, the trapezius and levator scapulae muscles twitched and jumped against my thumbs, a positive indication for trigger points.

A trigger point is a knot or nodule in a tight muscle. A trigger point can form as a result of repetitive actions, like faux painting walls all day, or by intense emotional or physical trauma causing muscles to contract and trap biochemicals inside.

Dr. Janet Travell, a pioneer of physical therapy, named these nodules 'trigger points'. Trigger points can cause severe pain at the area of the involved muscle, but they can also refer pain to other areas not directly associated with the muscle.

For example, a trigger point nodule in the trapezius muscle of the shoulder can refer pain up into the neck and head, causing neck pain and headaches. These referred pains make you think the problem is in your neck or your head, when it's really in the muscle in your shoulder. Dr. Travell was the personal physician of President John F. Kennedy, working to release the trigger points that were one of the causes of his frequent debilitating migraines.

True trigger points don't go away on their own,

they must have direct pressure applied to the exact point, long enough for the muscle fibers to release. Treating a trigger point will temporarily increase the pain, so, if you have a headache from a trigger point, pressing on the trigger point will make your head feel worse.

When the muscle knot has biochemistry, like hormones or waste products from a previous life trauma locked up inside of it, releasing the muscle knot, releases those old chemicals of emotion. Thus causing the patient to re-experience the ancient emotions, causing nausea, tears or anxiety, making you feel like crap, as though, the past event were happening now.

Christy had loads of trigger points creating a minefield of locked up pain. To help her, I had to navigate her traumatized soul. I had to release some of these knots before I could work on her neck.

She was so tense and guarded that I was afraid I just couldn't work on her.   But slowly, with gentle loving kindness, she began to trust me, just a little, but enough to allow the hot packs and the gentle massage to soften her armor. My heavy hot packs create a warm, womb like cocoon, inducing relaxation and comfort, even Christy found comfort from them.

I did what I could in that short first visit, but I recommended that she return for more work. It was a difficult session, since her degree of defensiveness had me weighing my every movement and word, being careful not to hit an emotional trigger, and driving her back into her fortress. She spat out a wise crack or barbed remark, whenever I got too close. To be honest, I really didn't expect her to return.

I was totally surprised, when the very next week, she called for another appointment.

This time, when she walked through the door, she actually seemed like a different person, lighter, brighter and genuinely happy to see me. It would be nice, I thought, if my work had such a profound effect, that removing a thorn from her paw, so to speak, had released a new lightness to her personality.

With a lilting, whimsical tone, she started to tell me about a vision that she just recently experienced. She often had visions. She said that, throughout her life, these visions helped her through difficult times or revealed events from her past or future. This particularly poignant vision was of a past life from long ago. She had been a man, a powerful warrior, a proud soldier. Her previous soldier self , she said, had during battle, become critically, horribly, wounded. Weak and near death, but through determination and fortitude, he fought his way through the forest to a small dusty village. Her, or rather, *His* injuries were so severe that no one dared touch him. They were all terrified of a badly wounded, dangerous, soldier.

Your only hope, they advised him, was to go to the

"Freak in the Grotto". She is very strange and bizarre, and lives all alone. The birds, bees, animals, and trees are her friends. She helps everyone, and everything, that comes to her door. Maybe she can help you. She's a crazy witch, but her magic is potent.

He slowly and painfully made his way to the edge of the village and out into the woods with brave desperation, not completely dead, but almost dead, he crawled through the brush. Hidden among the trees, he came upon a tiny, ivy covered, thatched roof, cottage.

With his last ounce of strength, he pounded fiercely on the thick wooden door. Collapsing on the threshold, he heard a gentle voice calling from inside. When the door was slowly opened, "It was you!," she said to me, "you were the freak in the grotto! And you were short then, too!"

I had been a short, kooky, wild woman, freak, and I saved his life. I felt the truth in her vision immediately. I honestly believed that we had that encounter way back then. Even today, I am still a freak, and she is still a battled scared warrior, fighting for survival.

Her vision allowed her to trust me, opening the doors to her guarded castle of pain. Truly believing that I could help her, she allowed me to do the deep and painful work needed to release the trigger points in her muscles. After that, her neck pain and headaches were greatly relieved. I saw her just a few times, but the effect was profound and she felt like a different person.

Months passed and Suzie and Christy eventually separated. Suzie was heartbroken. I'm sorry to say, I was not surprised. Christy, I thought, was not really long term relationship material. She was, in her love life and in our healthcare sessions, a runner, if you got too close.

Without the impetus of Christy, the parties stopped and the house calmed down. Joanie, however, the overly boyish work booted dyke, continued to live in the trailer in the front yard, a reminder of the exciting, but short lived episode.

One morning, a year or so later, I got a call from Suzie. She was very upset and said that Christy had called her, and she sounded insane. "More than usual?", I asked. "Yes!" she cried. "way more than usual! I was on the phone with her and I could hear her running in the street. She's jumping in front of cars, she's stopping them and yelling in the car windows, screaming at people, warning them that the aliens are going to take their children. She's screaming on the phone, telling me to run and prepare for a space invasion Armageddon!

We have to do something, please, she's going to get killed." Suzie begged, "Please come and help me, she says she'll only talk to you. She doesn't want to talk to me, only you."

What!? Why me, I thought. "Well," I said firmly, immediately giving in, "I won't go without you. I hardly know her and this is way above and beyond the call of duty. She lives half way to L.A."

So off we went. We got into Suzie's broken down, Volkswagen, rattle trap and drove down the freeway. We made our way down to where Christy was living in her mother's house. Christys' Mom, I learned, had recently died. I thought that losing her mom, may have been the trigger that sent her over the edge. Losing a mom is a devastating event. No matter how we feel about our moms, when they are gone, we feel the emptiness and pain of their absence. It could be, that her mom was the one who helped her remember to take her meds. She was definitely not on her meds that day!

As I got out of the car, I was confronted by a wired up, wise cracking, lunatic. Her eyes were wild and her actions were big and uncontrolled. Her beautiful blue eyes looked right through me, she wasn't focused on reality. She was on a different planet. Out on the front lawn strutting around like she ruled the world, she was still yapping and yelling and running into the street. She never stopped moving. After a long while, she seemed to slow down and began pacing in circles around the lawn.

Finally able to approach her I casually asked her, "What's going on, Christy?" She replied with a bunch of nonsense. I couldn't understand her, it was indecipherable gibberish. Suzie tried to get her into the house, but she wouldn't go. Hyperactive and manic, she kept saying something about aliens coming to get us all, and that we were all going to die. Then she took off, jogging out into the street and stopping cars. I ran after her and gently, but firmly, got her to leave the people and the cars alone.

Then, she started laughing and looking at me like it was all a huge joke. Trying to shepherd her to a safe spot, I told her that we should go inside. She pulled away from me, screaming that it wasn't safe. I had enough. I wasted no more time, I called the psychiatric swat team. I told them that, "yes, she was a danger to others", and that, "yes, she was a danger to herself." They said they'd be right over.

It seemed like 'right over' took forever. Finally, a large black station wagon with two big men pulled up in front. A police cruiser pulled in right behind them, and two overstuffed policemen with their hands resting on their holsters got out of their car.

The two burly counselors tried talking to her, trying to get her basic information. The birth date she gave them was off by about twenty years. They came to talk to me saying they couldn't do anything with her unless she voluntarily got into the vehicle. She hadn't broken any laws, and she couldn't be forced to commit herself to a program. So it came down to me.

I had to talk her into getting into that car, into giving them her right name and birthday, and to agree, in writing, to treatment. But, how? I tried speaking to her for awhile. It was like talking to a teenager. I've had experience talking to troublesome teens, so I talked to her like a mom. And then I spoke to her like the freak in the grotto.

I doubted that she would remember the vision, but the weird interaction caught her attention, and she connected.

I spoke to whatever molecule of the real Christy was bouncing around in there. "Remember me?" I said, "The freak in the grotto?" She laughed, she seemed to remember. Our eyes connected. The intense visionary connection was her truth. She gave me, the freak, a believable full name and birth date. And then, thank heaven, she signed the form.

She looked into my eyes, relying on my integrity. "Really?"she said, "Really, should I get into this car with these guys?"

"Yes," I said, "Yes, Please, you'll be fine. I promise you, you'll be fine."

And before she would move, she made it clear, "Okay", she said, "Okay, I'm trusting you. I'm trusting YOU."

As I guided her into the vehicle, I shook the stranger's hand, to whom I was entrusting, this war torn warrior from my past. I prayed to god that I was doing the right thing and that they could help her settle back down to reality.

Sitting in the back seat of the black paddy wagon, she turned to look at me through the window, she smiled, cocking her one eyebrow, as if to say, "Don't worry, I got this."

I was relieved, heart broken and exhausted. This

amazing, intensely talented young woman, was living a life of pain and anguish. If a Psychiatrist could get her back on the right meds, she would need to stay on them forever. I know mentally challenged people who function amazingly well when they were on their meds. Taking their meds faithfully allows them to lead a more normal life.

There are many highly intelligent and amazing people, like Christy, who live on the edge of insanity. The prospect is frightening for me. Imagine having a friend or loved one, just a breath away from going insane.

I've read where neurological dysfunction can be a result of generalized inflammation. People with a propensity for depression, anxiety, obsessive compulsive, or bipolar disorder, will become more susceptible to dysfunction when inflammation sets up in their system. One way to help avoid excessive inflammation is to regularly supplement the diet with natural anti-inflammatories. For example, fish oil, curcumin, boswellia, and echinacea, if taken every day, will help reduce inflammation in the entire body.

Reducing inflammation will improve physical and mental health enormously. But, on top of that, the newest information states that reducing SIBO, (remember from Chapter 6) may help to reduce symptoms of obsessive-compulsive disorder, anxiety, depression and amazingly enough, schizophrenia.

Remember, the protocol is to try to kill off the

bad bacteria overgrowth in the small intestine with a combination of myrrh and artemsinin, then rebuild with probiotics.

Eliminating sugars, refined carbohydrates, and fried foods, is also imperative if this treatment protocol is going to work. You will have to go through several cycles of treatment, consisting of four to five days of Myrrh and Artemisinin, followed by seven to ten days of probiotics. Sugar and simple carbohydrates must be eliminated during the entire time, and hopefully, result in eliminating sugar from the diet forever.

In my experience, keeping connections with family and friends allows patients to be monitored in case they decide to take a vacation from their medication. We can't live their lives for them, but we can check on them, be vigilant for them, and be aware when they are struggling. I believe in holistic treatments, but also in taking advantage of medical advances, including psychotropic drugs, when our lives can be miraculously saved or improved by them.

At this time in my life, my dear friend, Suzie, lives far away, but spiritually, she is a breath away. I am never alone because my friend is always here in my heart (and on Facebook).

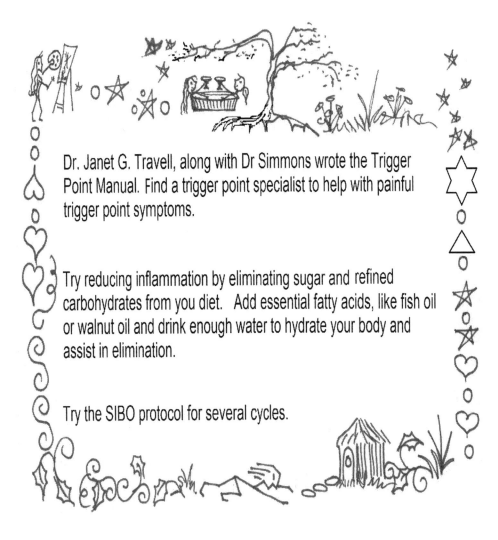

Dr. Janet G. Travell, along with Dr Simmons wrote the Trigger Point Manual. Find a trigger point specialist to help with painful trigger point symptoms.

Try reducing inflammation by eliminating sugar and refined carbohydrates from you diet. Add essential fatty acids, like fish oil or walnut oil and drink enough water to hydrate your body and assist in elimination.

Try the SIBO protocol for several cycles.

Chapter 11
The tap on the shoulder

I, sometimes, find myself unable to handle just one more thing. When that thing turns up, I do what we all do, I ignore it. It might be the same thing that I've been ignoring all my life or it could be something new, confusing, and the last straw for my overburdened body and brain. So, if that's the case, I consciously ignore it. While my subconscious mind is busy, trying to find a deep, dark, nook or cranny, to bury the little nuisance away somewhere, to be either forgotten, or worse, allowed to fester.

The offensive issue is hidden, all in an effort to guard us from unwanted pain and suffering. This unsettled emotion is lying in wait at a subconscious level. Eventually, when the time is right, it begins to send out messages that something is wrong, and now, might be a good time to deal with it. When the issue erupts as pain, that's the point when this hidden emotion has officially transformed into psychosomatic pain.

When this psychosomatic pain starts bubbling up to the surface, the first thing it will do is tap us on the shoulder. "Hey, I'm here, remember me?." If we choose to ignore the tap, the next time our body will tap us a little harder, "Hey you!, Pay attention, this is important." Then a lot harder, and then finally, tired of being ignored, it will hit us with a two by four.

"Hey Stupid, wake up, you got a problem."

If we are wise enough to seek help during the tap on the shoulder stage, we might be able to work through the issue with a close friend or loved one, or maybe even, a caring health care provider. But, choosing to ignore the symptom, or deciding instead, to go to a doctor who provides only drugs or surgery, thereby ignoring the emotional component, the problem will persist and fester. Drugs or surgery won't relieve it, and you're left with unremitting chronic pain.

Only through loving and caring can we overcome the emotional cause behind the physical pain. Sometimes it's not easy to find a friend or loved one willing to go through such a process with us, and really, the lack of such a person in our life can be the whole problem. In that case, seek out a counselor, spiritual adviser, or healthcare practitioner, and then work toward making friends. Look in the local paper for community activities or join a group.

As a chiropractor, I not only adjust the spine, I listen and care for the whole person, body and soul. I touch people who don't get touched, I listen to people who need to be heard, and I love people who need love.

Some people don't like to be touched. For some, touch has been an assault and to be touched is scary. When I touch those people, I can feel their entire body tense up. They guard themselves against even the gentlest massage or embrace. They want to be loved, but they can't help their fearful reaction to it.

As I search for the troubled area, screaming to be rescued, sometimes the person will say, "I know what it is." They will sometimes tell me that it's their husband, their kid, their job, or even their mother. And then they will share with me the unique personal stories of heartache, abuse, anguish, or pain.

Being on the outside looking in, I can sometimes see what they can't. If they can't see it, it may be that they don't want to see it, or they're not ready to face it. I have to be careful not to say things that they can't handle, so sometimes, I can't say anything at all. If a person is not ready to see the truth, pushing the truth in their face could freak them out and make them feel worse. It's not for me to rob them of their destiny and deny them their life lessons.

I won't push truth into their face, but I can gently ask questions and open doors. If they feel it's time to walk through the door, then we can do it together. If not, then we just work with their body, help relieve the pain, and help them get back to work, or play or whatever matters to them the most.

To work with the mind body connection, we need to trust and be comfortable with each other. I can tell them my story, or stories that I've heard that relate to them, or their situation. Relating these stories lets them see that other people have had these types of problems too. That's what this book is for. If you recognize yourself or someone you love in these stories, maybe the remedies will help you or them overcome the burden and move forward into love and light. Whatever you or a loved one may be going through, it's not so terrible, when you realize that you're not the only one who's had to deal with a situation like it. There are very few problems that are truly unique.

I've had patients burst into tears after a chiropractic adjustment. Just the adjustment can release the locked up emotions, along with the painful mis-alignment. The tears come from deep within, and they're not from pain, but from chemicals of emotions, hormones trapped in tight muscles and body parts. These ancient emotions may have been trapped and locked up for years. The adjustment can trigger a physical release accompanied by an emotional release, similar to the emotional vomiting Roberta experienced in Peru.

Sometimes, with this type of emotional baggage, we can let go of the suitcase, without having to look at what's inside. If we release the chemicals, the ancient event just releases along with it. After we metabolize the waste products, we just piss it all out. That's why it's important to drink lots of water. There's lots of stuff that just needs to be pissed out.

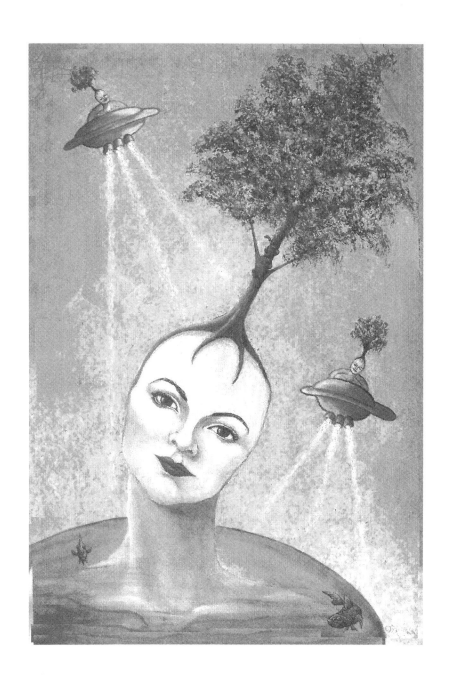

Healing Heads from Outer Space

Chapter 12
Guess who!

I have a website because every professional has a website. I thought it would be fun to post pictures of myself, at wild and crazy Luna parties. Inspiring, as well as entertaining. My favorite picture is the one of me in a big, long, curly, red, wig and steam punk outfit. I love that one. No one knows it's me until later, when the pics show up on my website.

In addition to being a chiropractor, I'm an artist. I also post my paintings up on my website. I paint my personal truths, life lessons bought and paid for. Lessons that I have learned through painful periods of growth and enlightenment. My personal truth series of paintings are representations of: Emergence of personal power, Allowance of knowledge and wisdom, Release of holdings, and Transcendence by traveling to the power of the full moon on the howl of a wolf. These are major life lessons for me. Concepts that I have set to canvas as a way of confirming my vision. One of the biggest lessons I've learned is that wisdom and enlightenment often come with struggle and pain. My web address is listed at the end of this book, if your interested in examining my artwork.

My -do it yourself- website came with the usual conservative banal lingo. But, with my amateur customization, it now represents my more flamboyant, eccentric, personal style. I include photos of my truth series paintings along with pictures from fun and exciting Luna costume parties. I post my office hours along with my phone number and spiritual philosophy.

I created my website for kicks, but once in a while, I actually get a patient notification from it. My e-mail account notifies me when a new patient would like an appointment. It's surprising to me that someone would choose me from my crazy website. It seems like such an impersonal way to choose a health care provider, especially when the website looks more like a joke than a serious representation of a business.

I prefer phone calls from new patients. I like to hear the timbre of their voice. It exudes the essence of their personality, and allows my subconscious mind to do the "blink" thing. I don't check my e-mail regularly, therefore, it could take days for me to reply. Luckily, this time, I noticed the message right away and replied with a time for him to come in. Through the miracle of cyberspace, his appointment was confirmed.

Nice surprise and right on time, this really handsome, tall, Alaskan made, hunk of a guy, limps through the door. Dressed for the forest, he radiated strength and vitality. He seemed quite perfect in every way, except for a persistent hitch in his get-along. He told me honestly that he'd already seen a few different chiropractors, and his pain in the butt, just wasn't going away. He presented with diffused pain along his low back and pointed pain in the center of his buttox.

First thing I think, as I sat listening to him explain his condition, is that the problem is probably with his Psoas muscle. The Psoas is the major postural muscle of the pelvic girdle and one of the most common causes for low back pain. It originates at the head of the femur, then runs under the inguinal ligament, and finally anchors on the lumbar spine, right in the area of his low back, where he was pressing with his fist. This muscle can cause the spine to twist and/or compress, both reactions causing severe low back pain or sciatica. Prolonged sitting, at the computer, riding in a plane, driving in a car, or just plopping down in front of the TV, allows our Psoas to become short, fat, stiff and tight. Thus causing one of the most common symptoms of severe low back pain.

The first thing I had him do, even before touching him, was to do some Psoas stretches, which are similar to the warrior pose in yoga.

Lunge forward keeping the back leg straight and the front knee bent, body 90 degrees to the floor, focusing on the front of the hip of the back leg. (See illustration 1)

Stretching these muscles gets them warmed up for the pain relieving adjustment. Stretching this muscle is the only way to lengthen and loosen it, preventing recurring low back pain. It's one of the stretches that everyone should do every day. When stretching, always stop if it causes or increases pain.

As he was stretching, I asked him if he just picked my name off the internet. He said no, and that he was at a party the other night and asked if any one knew of a good chiropractor and three people said my name. He felt that that was a clear sign to call me. That explained why he contacted me, in spite of my zany website.

After stretching both sides twice, I directed him to lie down, nose in the hole, on my chiropractic table. I checked his leg length, and hip height, and placed the usual hot packs on his back. Then, I stretched his quads.

The quadriceps, located at the front of the thigh, are another postural muscle group that should be stretched every day. Stretching his quadriceps muscles caused major spasms in his calves. If your calf muscles spasm during stretches, or if calf spasms wake you up at night, like a "Charlie horse", that's a sign of calcium deficiency, and I suggest that you take supplements.

I questioned him about his hydration, electrolytes, calcium and essential fatty acid supplementation, all of which are essential for optimum muscle health and function. He said that he was so busy going back and forth to Alaska, because his beloved mom had recently passed away, and he had to clean out her house, and prepare it for rental. He just didn't have time to follow his usual health and supplement routine.

He was overwhelmed, and had forgotten to take care of himself. It's a common situation. We get so busy and tired that we forget to take care of ourselves. But, that's the time when we need it the most. If we don't take the time to care for ourselves, we will regret it. My mother always used to say, "Ya gotta take care of yourself, cause nobody else will." He had tried to do some stretching, but his back was hurting so bad, he had to stop.

Aside from stretching the Psoas and Quadriceps every day for the rest of his life, I recommended fish oil and calcium magnesium supplementation. I recommend cod liver oil supplements, being that they supply essential fatty acids, along with vitamin A and D. I told him the brand I use comes from the Norwegian Sea (I like to stay away from fish oil that may have been exposed to Fukashima waters). He said, "Oh yeah, when I was a kid in Alaska my mom used to give me cod liver oil every day." There was never enough sun light in Alaska for his body to produce sufficient amounts of vitamin D and his mom knew what to do.

Vitamin D is essential for our overall good health. It regulates the absorption of calcium, and helps prevent heart disease, cancer, diabetes, and dementia. It is also essential for our immune system to fight infections. So many people are avoiding the sun for fear of skin cancer that vitamin D deficiency is very common. If your not getting at least 20 minutes of sun a day, then you need to supplement your diet with vitamin D.

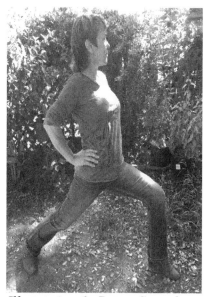

Illustration 1: Psoas Stretch, Always do both sides. Hold each side for the count of 20 seconds. remember to breath. Feel the stretch, stop if it causes pain.

When he got up to leave he said he felt a lot better, but he had one last thing to say. "I don't want to say anything bad about any of the other chiropractors, because they were all good, but none of the other doctors I've seen, mentioned hydration, nutrition, or stretching. I need to get back to my stretching program and back on those supplements that my mother used to give me."

I always recommend an organic food source vitamin and mineral supplement with an extra supplement of essential fatty acids, to be taken every day for the rest of our lives.

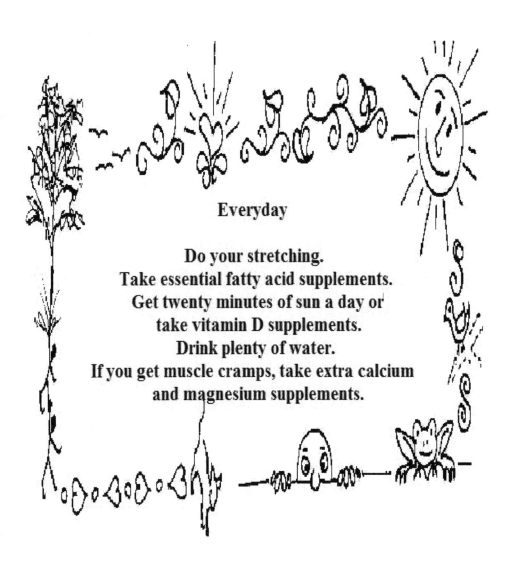

Everyday

Do your stretching.
Take essential fatty acid supplements.
Get twenty minutes of sun a day or
take vitamin D supplements.
Drink plenty of water.
If you get muscle cramps, take extra calcium
and magnesium supplements.

Chapter 13
The post-nuptial agreement

My friend, Victoria, is so much fun. Vibrant and luscious, she was raised in the farming region of Pennsylvania, where the fresh air and the chilly winter gave her the complexion of an Ivory soap girl. Am I the only person who remembers the Ivory Soap girl commercial? Lovely, healthy skin with rosy cheeks and a smile as bright as the California sun. Like a true beauty queen, her thick, wavy, blonde hair, bounces when the rest of her bounces into my office. Her cheeks dimple and her eyes twinkle, when she smiles, she looks just like a slim Mrs. Santa Claus. She's one of the nicest people I've ever met in all my life.

Victoria grew up, like me, on Disney fairy tales. Prince charming would seek us out and take us home to his palace on the hill. Victoria's Prince came in from California, swept her off her Pennsylvania feet, and transported her to the other side of the country, away from her friends, family and hometown that she had known all her life.

Happy as a little clam, Victoria settled down to a fantasy lifestyle that included a lovely home, a hard working prince charming, and California sunshine every day. Shortly after they married and settled, Victoria became pregnant with their first child. She was happy with Ross as her husband, but he worked a lot and she felt like she never saw him. Pregnant in a new town, she felt all alone, and complained that he worked too much.

"Do you want a buddy, or do you want food to eat?" he scolded her. "I just want to spend a little more time together" she meekly replied, "I'm lonely."

Eventually her little bundle of boy was born. She was consumed with motherhood. Ross could have taken some time off from work, to help with the infant and recovering mom, but he didn't. So Victoria was left alone, far away from her mom and support system.

Two years later, the second baby arrived and then she had two boys to shower her love upon. Ross was usually MIA, and almost never came home before dark. At least with the babies, she wasn't alone. She'd made a good catch with Ross, but she wondered if all the stuff was worth her loneliness. Whenever she complained about his absence, he reminded her what his absence was able to provide. She didn't argue, she did love her beautiful house and she wanted the best for her children.

The business did well during the first few years of their marriage, and when the second little boy was born, Ross came home with some paperwork for her to sign.

"What's this for?" she asked her dear husband. He told her not to worry, it was just business. Not giving it another thought, and thoroughly trusting in

Ross, she signed where she was told to and put the contract out of her mind.

Our beautiful girl from Pennsylvania was a wonderful wife and mother, but the more money they made, the lonelier she became. Her children were growing and entering school and she was once again, left home alone. She spent her mornings cooking and cleaning the fabulous new mansion that Ross had bought for them. But, it was further from town and at the top of the hill.

She had a cleaning lady, Maria, come to the house twice a week but, there was really nothing much to clean. Victoria kept the house immaculate. She just really appreciated the company. Maria taught her Spanish, and they became friends.

She had thought, when she first met Ross, that having money and a big house in California was going to be a dream come true. Her fairy tale life was having children and a loving husband. She found as the kids grew up, she was left alone in a cold empty shell of a house.

She called my office, after having sat cross legged on the cold, concrete garage floor. She'd spent hours working on costumes for the boys' school program. Her artistic passion and obsession with excellence led her to sit for hours, every day, perfecting their costumes and the backdrop for their performance. She didn't stop to eat, or drink, or some nights, even to make dinner.

She came to me complaining of low back pain.

The root chakra at the base of the spine is the foundation for back support, but also the energetic foundation for hearth and home, family and finances.

I love seeing her. She's fun and bubbly with an eccentric artist's soul. The first thing we do, after we hug, is stretch. I do them with her. The Psoas stretch, Quad stretch, Hamstring stretch, and the Piriformis stretch, then I force her to drink water.

After the stretching session, she is already feeling better. It's amazing what a little bit of stretching and hydration can do.

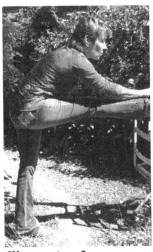

Illustration 2:
Hamstring Stretch.
Stretching t he back of
the thigh. Do both
sides. Hold to the
count of 20. Breath.

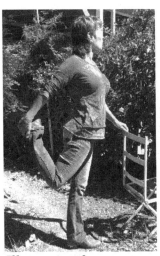

Illustration 3:
Quadriceps Stretch .
Stretching the front of
the thigh. Do both
sides. Hold to the count
of 20. Breath

One day I start to realize that I'm seeing her so often, I begin to wonder what is else is going on. I get the feeling that it's more than just sitting on the concrete floor. Maybe this condition has an emotional component. And, maybe, she is ignoring the true problem, that is now, just tapping her on the shoulder. If she continues to ignore the warning, the next step, remember, is like being hit with a two by four. When we discuss her life, she admits to being unhappy. She's been so lonely for so long, that instead of cheerful, she's miserable. She can't seem to connect with her husband anymore. He doesn't talk to her, but then, she admits, he never did.

"I just thought that, that's how men are, my mother always said that men really don't talk much." she explained.

It's common for men to be taciturn, but Ross wasn't just quiet, he was never there. The more money they made, the more obsessed Ross and the boys became with sports cars, boats and man toys of all kinds. He spent the evenings in his garage, and the weekends out playing with his boys and their toys. It seemed to Victoria that he loved his stuff more than her. She felt like a maid, only Maria, the real maid, was happier with her tiny house and family than Victoria was with her mansion and cars. She had a spectacular house and pool, a fancy car and luxurious toys, but we all know that stuff doesn't make you happy.

She missed the old days, when the kids were small, and they played together all the time. No surprise, the boys preferred sports cars and boats, way more than being with mom. Children are like that, it's normal as they get older, that we're not their preferred playmates anymore. They're supposed to branch out on their own, preparing to leave the nest. But it's still painful to watch our children leave, especially when we've structured our whole life around them.

I encouraged her to find an outlet for her passion and artistry. She loved to travel and they had plenty of money, so she suggested to Ross that they go traveling. Ross had to work, couldn't leave the business, and had better things to do. She tried begging, but that got her nowhere, So, lonely and hurting, she decided to go alone.

She found her passion, taking lovely, romantic, photos of historic sites, all over Spain and Italy. By finding just the right angle or focus, she turned peeling, cracking, crumbling, ruins, into lovely, moving, masterpieces. With her artistic genius, her one woman show, in the local coffee house, sold out the first day.

Wherever she went, she missed her husband and her sons. Unfortunately, her husband and sons didn't miss her.

She plastered a dimpled smile on her pretty face and carried on. The more she pretended to be happy, the more she actually became happy. It has been concluded through studies, that just the act of smiling can improve your mood. She was rediscovering her joy. She learned to speak Spanish from Maria, so,

Spain was her favorite place. Barcelona is an artists' paradise, with the Park Guell and the Cathedral Sagrada Familia, it's a constant inspiration. Her pigeon Spanish, or Spanglish, was endearing and along with her natural beauty she had more friends in Spain than she had in California. Good cheer has a language all it's own and she was, once again, fluent in good cheer.

She met so many interesting people, but one Spanish couple in particular became her best friends. They were almost young enough to be her children, and she was thrilled to be in their company. She was their mothers age, but they said that their mother wasn't that much fun.

One day they brought their father along. The four of them had great excursions and adventures throughout Spain. Spanish people seem to have more time for walking, talking, living, and playing. Some of the things, we Americans, don't seem to have much time for. Her new friends treated her like family and she always brought them exquisite gifts from America.

They began writing letters back and forth, keeping in touch, until finally, just Victoria and the dad, Antonio, were pen pals. He had trouble writing in English, so most of his letters were in Spanish.

One day, she brought a particularly long letter, written in Spanish, down to the coffee shop. She had a Spanish speaking friend, Sergio, who agreed to translate the letter for her. He read the letter through and then he read it again. He paused and looked thoughtful, and then tried to translate it to her. After a minute, he put the letter down.

"Victoria," he said, "this man loves you."

"Oh yes," she giggled, "he's so nice, I love him too."

"No, Victoria, he doesn't love you like that. It's not a friendship kind of love. He really, really, loves you, like, loves you, loves you. Get it? He is in love with you." Sergio pressured her with the truth.

Victoria was stunned. Dumbfounded, she stepped back and put her hand to her throat. "NO, no, not really," she said, "Really?"

"Yes, really." Sergio assured her.

And, that, was when everything changed for Victoria.

I'd see her whenever she came home from one of her trips, or when she had overdone it with one of her projects, forgetting once again to stretch regularly. She usually brought me a wonderful gift from her travels. She's always been so generous and kind, plus she has great taste.

More confused than ever, she was in love and not with her husband. Her honesty led her to confess her feelings to her husband, which of course, led to a huge angry fight. Not surprising, it wasn't pretty.

Remember that contract she signed fifteen years ago when her children were babies. Well, it turned out, it was a post-nuptial agreement. When she signed that contract she was young, vulnerable, naive and trusting, and had just given birth. She had done what he asked, and fifteen years later, the true diabolical nature of the request was clear. If she ever left him, she would leave broke. She was a heartsick mess. Young, and totally in love, when she married her handsome, young husband, she now came to realize, that all of his manipulations were fueled by greed. She had always, cared for Ross, the kids, the house, and his business, for sixteen years. She deserved to be treated better than this.

The contract left her over a barrel. Ross was willing to keep their marriage together, but she would have to give up her visits to Spain, along with her Spanish lover. Ross said that he still loved her, but things for her would have to change. Things for Ross would stay the same, in that he would still go out and about, working and playing as he liked, and she would once again be left behind, in her lonely mansion on the hill.

Agreeing to try and save her marriage, she began to go along with him on the boat, but she didn't like his friends, and there were lots of young women along, all of them drinking and partying. She longed for Antonio and found herself needing to make a difficult decision. Money or love.

Victoria adored her children and her husband. She worked desperately to win Ross' love, but he just didn't have any love to give. His drunken father handled young Ross with cold angry abuse and heavy handedness. Ross never healed from his childhood abuse and having never been loved, he never learned how.

Victoria chose love.

Blind with rage, Ross cut her off from everything he could. She had married Ross when she was just eighteen, and was unfamiliar with being all on her own. She needed a job. Her bubbly personality got her a job as an Activities Director and she was perfect for it. The money she earned was nothing compared to the money she was used to having, and slowly she learned to cope and economize. They went to court and the judge honored the post-nuptial agreement to a point, but he felt that Victoria deserved her personal property of jewels, clothes, automobile, and a stipend for upkeep, until she was able to find a way to more comfortably support herself.

They shared custody of the teenage boys, but the boys, not surprisingly, preferred to spend their time in the huge family home playing with their games, and their dad. Without Victoria, the warmth had gone out of the home, but the money was there, and that was enough to keep them happy for awhile.

Her American divorce was pretty quick. The jewelry, which the judge had allotted her, was a treasure trove. Looking to sell the more exquisite pieces, she laid them out on the table to photograph them. It was exciting to see, touch, and try on, the dazzling jewels. My favorite piece from the collection, was a beautiful 14 kt. Gold rope, studded with sapphires and diamonds.   That one bracelet was so heavy,   the gold alone was worth a fortune. She got a bundle for that bracelet.   It was a good thing too because she needed the money to live. Nice trailers around here in the Luna area, go for big bucks, plus space rent, and she wanted a home of her own.   Thank god for the jewelry. She showed me a ring that she had chosen for her Christmas present one year, it was gold and platinum with a diamond the size of jawbreaker.   That huge rock, symbolized their marriage -- expensive, but cold and heartless. Selling that ring was the final closing curtain to her marriage.

Every few months, she would show up at my door, complaining of low back pain. "I hurt so bad! I think I have bone cancer!" she wailed. "You said that last time," I reminded her, "and you know, you didn't have bone cancer. You were just out of alignment."

The low back pain had come from the core of her unhappy marriage, but now, the pain was more severe with her broken family, estranged children, and total lack of financial support.

So, I do my thing: I heat her, stretch her, and adjust her. Abracadabra! Her pain is gone. "Looks like you don't have bone cancer" I said "because, you know, I can't cure bone cancer.   The low back is where the root Chakra for home, family and finances is located. When that Chakra is negatively activated, it causes low back pain. Please try to meditate, maybe do some journaling, drink more water and *Stretch*!!!"

Victoria had made her choice, love over money. The two lovebirds, found out that, although Victoria's American divorce was a financial disaster, divorce in Spain was even more emotionally grueling and financially devastating. The Spanish wife was way beyond pissed off. She was poisonously enraged and determined to make Antonio suffer.

Antonio had already been suffering for years. He refused to be bitter and embraced the new found love in his life. Antonio and Victoria chose love and happiness. They might be poor in pocket, but they were rich in their hearts, hearth, and spirits.

With the money she got from selling her jewelry, Victoria bought a small mobile home. The place was a dowdy fixer upper, but Victoria's gifts transformed the dull, outdated, double wide coach, into a lovely Tuscany Style warm retreat. She painted murals of Italian landscapes on the walls and festooned the elegant furniture with lush Italian tapestries. The fabrics, colors and textures, filled the home, creating a warm romantic nest for her and her beloved Antonio.

On his first visit to America, I spoke to him about the turn his life had taken. He said that, meeting Victoria had actually saved his life. He was dying of misery before he met her, and now, his heart was bursting with love and joy. He called her his Cappuccino. They spent four month together every year, when she went to visit him in Spain from

America. But, until they were married, she couldn't stay. She had to come home, get a job, and finish raising her boys.

Antonio's wife continued to make his life a living hell. It took years to get the divorce and then his wife got everything, all the assets, and all the money.

No one could blame his wife for being pissed off and vengeful. But, oddly enough, she found a lover almost right away. Looking back, Antonio was so unhappy because he and his wife no longer shared their life with each other. It turns out he worked while she played. Only she was playing with someone else. She had another wealthy, handsome, lover all along. Once the divorce began she moved into a luxurious home with him. She had no use for the family home that she had shared with Antonio. She didn't need it, she just didn't want him to have it.

Dear Antonio and his Cappuccino continued to struggle. Every year, she would get a leave of absence from her job and go to Spain. And every year, Antonio would take his vacation in America. They went from the tiny Spanish apartment to her little mobile home in California. Their circumstances so very different from their much more affluent past.

I've often wondered if there were regrets. She had lived in a mansion with expensive cars, and luxuries, and now she lived in a trailer park. Antonio was slaving away with none of his previous family comforts, no money, and an angry ex-wife.   If they were having second thoughts, it didn't show. Whenever I saw them together, they looked cozy and happy.

It took three and half years for the Spanish court to grant Antonio a divorce. He was still required to give his ex-wife all his money and she was granted his ancestral family home.

Antonio and Victoria were married in Spain and again in California.   They continued to live separately, working at their jobs, and trying to make ends meet. Victoria wanted them to live in America. Antonio would live anywhere. Here or there, home is where the heart is, and Victoria was his heart.

I almost never see Victoria in my office anymore. She exemplifies a basic truth of life – money cannot buy happiness. She has finally found true love, and found the courage to surrender to it.

There are no regrets for her. She is happy and in love. A love that is rarely found, and so filled with romance. If I didn't love them both so much,   I would be jealous.

Last time I saw her, she told me the news. The Spanish court had granted Antonio possession of his family home.   My dear friend, and her adoring husband, would be leaving us to start a new chapter in their lives. This new adventure will begin in Spain.   I've been invited to visit.   I hope she stretches, drinks water, and besides blissfully sleeping next to her handsome Spanish lover every night, I hope she laughs a lot!

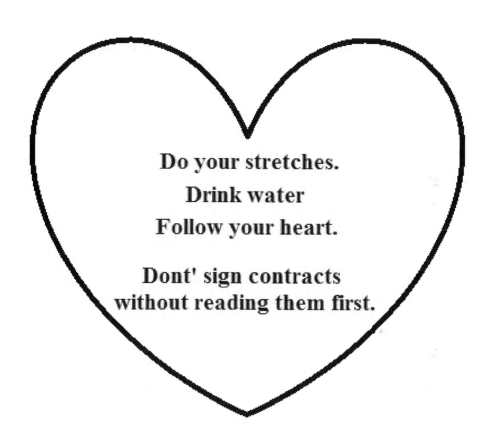

Do your stretches.
Drink water
Follow your heart.

Dont' sign contracts
without reading them first.

Chapter 14
Fix me, but don't touch me

Decades ago, when my Chiropractic office was still in downtown, one of my very first patients was an intelligent, but terrified young woman with a lovely, curly haired, baby girl in tow.

Before agreeing to come see me, she wanted a promise that I would work on her with out actually touching her.

"Yup," I said, "I can do that."

She'd been to a lot of different doctors and was tired of being in pain. Her previous chiropractor had been a little rough with her, but she was still hopeful that another, more gentle chiropractor, could help.

Actually, I get that a lot. There are a few people, who have had bad experiences with chiropractors, and, as a result, will never go to another chiropractor, ever again. However, we all know that if a person has a bad experience with an MD, they just go to another MD., and try again. They don't swear off medical doctors, like they do chiropractors.

We poor chiropractors are all dumped into the same bucket, as though we are all the same. But, we're not. There are as many different techniques and philosophies as there are rocks in a stream.

The two main categories are force and non-force. I use a combination of many different techniques, along with a variety of massage applications, and nutritional counseling. I work personally and carefully with the body, mind, and spirit.

As a result of my diversified and caring approach, many of my patients recommend me to their friends and loved ones, many who may have had a bad experience with chiropractic in the past. I tell them right off, *I may not be able to "fix" you, but I won't hurt you.*

Kelly showed up at my office with her young daughter anxiously clutching her hand. Both gals looked suspicious and frightened. Her history included a terrifying diagnosis of Multiple Sclerosis, recently given to her by a local MD. The condition was supposedly diagnosed by a barrage of medical tests.

As a young mother, she was looking forward to having a long happy life, proudly watching her baby girl grow into a woman. The prospect of an uncertain, slow, crippling future, which MS carries with it, was an emotional burden that was more crippling than the diagnosis. More terrified of MS than of me, she was willing to give me a chance to work on her.

First of all, let me be clear, I can't cure MS, I can't *cure* anything. I'm just here to unblock and unlock the electromagnetic circuits and channels of your body to allow our inherent, innate, healing energy to flow through freely, and foster our recovery.

All of the systems in our body are related. Our

spiritual, physical, and emotional bodies are intertwined, forming one big, happy, living, loving, triangle of life. What affects our spirit, can and does affect anything and everything else in our lives. Getting a gut reaction, can make you sick to your stomach. Someone being a pain in the neck, can cause you to have a pain in the neck. Experiencing a broken heart can cause a heart attack.

I remember hearing the story of Carrie Fisher and Debbie Reynolds. Debbie's beloved daughter, Carrie Fisher, died of a heart attack, and one day later, her mother, Debbie Reynolds, died of heartbreak. It actually has a name, it's called Takotsubo syndrome, it means heartbreak syndrome, and it can cause arrhythmia, palpitations, heart attack and death.

Getting back to Kelly, I convinced her to lie on the table and let me palpate her spine, assessing her spinal alignment. So, actually, she did let me touch her, but she didn't want me 'cracking' her and I understood why.

I could feel quite a few blocked areas that were impeding the flow of energy, or Life Chi, that would normally run through her body. The most gentle low force technique that I use is called an activator. It's a small mechanical device that delivers a directed high velocity, low force impulse. People call it a clicker. It sounds like a staple gun and reminds me of a mini-jack hammer. The activator force is strategically directed to the misaligned spine and extremity joints. This technique is especially useful with people who don't want to be touched or who are extremely sensitive. That's all I used on her for the first few weeks and it helped.

The more we worked together, the more she began to trust me. Eventually, I was able to do some muscle work and manual manipulations. Since the activator instrument was the main tool that I used to correct her mis-alignments, technically, I worked on her without touching her.

The doctors had told her that along with MS, she had leaky gut syndrome, which was causing her indigestion and bloating. Actually, all the symptoms that she was complaining of, that led to her diagnosis of Multiple Sclerosis, could have been caused by leaky gut syndrome.

Leaky gut syndrome can effect all areas of your body, not just your gut. When properly functioning, the gut, composed of our stomach and small and large intestines, comprise a neurologically functioning second brain. The brain in our gut works in tandem with the brain in our skull.

There are many causes of intestinal inflammation, for instance, too much sugar, stress, alcohol, caffeine, drugs, genetically modified foods, or toxins. The gut lining acts as a barrier to unwanted molecules. When that lining is damaged or inflamed, it weakens, and enemies of the body get in. These enemies can be undigested food particles, yeast, toxins, or bad bacteria. We need bacteria in our gut, but we need the good strains of bacteria not the bad ones. The inflamed gut lining and leaky gut syndrome can cause bloating, gas, constipation, headaches, fatigue, depression, skin eruptions, rashes, weight gain, and back pain. Kelly had many of these symptoms, which along with some testing, led her doctor to diagnose her with MS.

My examination revealed that her third lumbar vertebrae was rotated causing pain, weakness, and digestive discomfort. We worked on many areas of her spine, but the lumbar spine was the area that gave the most relief. Eventually the pain, weakness, and digestive discomforts went away.

Kelly continues to follow a moderately restricted diet. She abstains from alcohol, gluten, non-organic foods, sugar, and highly processed foods. She also supplements with probiotics, which supplies the good bacteria that we want in our intestines. She also takes digestive enzymes whenever she eats, and she includes kefir, yoghurt, turmeric as an anti-inflammatory, and licorice root to regulate the adrenal gland and balance cortisol production. And last, but not least, especially for leaky gut, she drinks bone broth, which is amazing for healing the intestinal tract. You can get organic bone broth already prepared from several sources online, at your local health food store, or you can make it yourself. I recommend it heartily for improving the health and vitality of the gut.

Twenty years has passed since the day Kelly first walked through my door, and to this day, she remains free from M.S. The diagnosis was obviously in error, but the fear and stress it created in her life could have killed her. Not to mention, what the consequence of an unnecessary treatment could have done to her. I have heard of a diagnosis sending people to their graves, whether it was in error or not. I have also heard of the chemical cure being worse that the disease.

Luckily, my dear friend Kelly was spared whatever drugs or treatments, that were currently in vogue, for the horrible diagnosis that she was given. She is actually quite healthy and robust. She was able to be an active and involved mother throughout her daughter's life, and was there to witness her lovely, curly headed girl graduating with high academic honors from Berkeley.

We are both very proud of our girl.

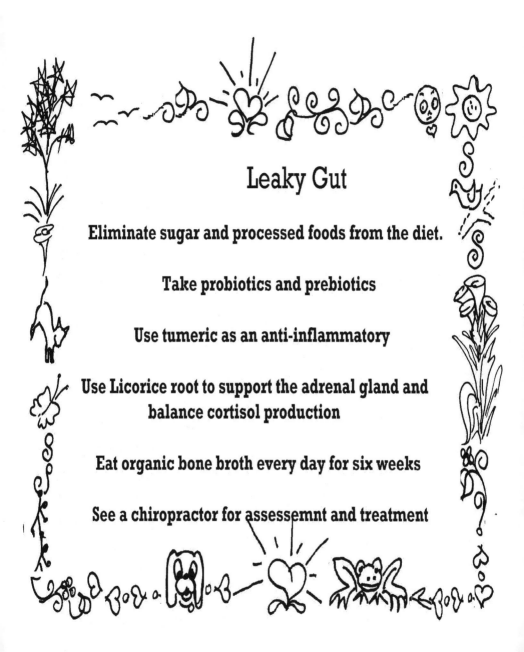

Leaky Gut

Eliminate sugar and processed foods from the diet.

Take probiotics and prebiotics

Use tumeric as an anti-inflammatory

Use Licorice root to support the adrenal gland and balance cortisol production

Eat organic bone broth every day for six weeks

See a chiropractor for assessemnt and treatment

Chapter 15
Too many red flags

Joel came in as a new patient. He was in his mid-fifties, a well dressed, well-spoken, slightly rotund man, complaining of low back pain. I love a well dressed man and Joel had great clothes. His suit was fitted, and flattering for his slightly heavy physique. Well mannered with a clean shaven face and expensive hair cut, he reminded me of the detective from the Agatha Christie movie, Murder on the Orient Express.

Joel said that he had been going to another chiropractor for quite some time, but had felt no relief.

Right away, that's a red flag.

"You've been seeing another chiropractor for months with no relief? Have you been to a medical doctor?" I asked. "I tried to get in," he replied, but they couldn't see me for a couple of weeks, so I decided to go the natural route." "Do you get regular check ups?" He answered me, by saying, that he doesn't like doctors, and he hadn't been in a while. Another red flag.

"Well, that's fine," I lied, " let me check you out."

When I had him down on my table, I started assessing his low back. I noticed that there were several reasons why his low back could be hurting. His hip was tilted backwards and his lower lumbar spine was twisted. I couldn't understand why it would still be so bad with all the chiropractic care this guy had been getting. But, patients don't always tell you the truth. Maybe he really hadn't seen his regular chiropractor for awhile.

Low back pain can have many causes, such as: wrenching muscles from golf or jogging, sitting too long at a desk, or overdoing it at the gym. There are also many diseases that can affect the bones.

So Joel, I discover, doesn't go to the gym, he doesn't play golf or sports of any kind. I see so many low back injuries from Golf that I just want to say right here that Golf is a really common way to twist your low back. It's important to get some help with your form when you take up golf, the proper swing is very important in avoiding injury.

In our computer driven society, almost every one I see, sits too long in front of their computer. This is the number one most common way to induce constant low back pain and poor posture. Sitting all day at a desk, never getting up to stretch, and never getting regular exercise, that was Joel's routine.

I recommend that everyone who sits at their computer for more than fifty minutes at a time, get up every hour and stretch. The psoas, the hamstring, and the quadricep stretch for a minimum of three minutes. You can actually do all three and make a difference in your health in three minutes.

How's your mattress? How do you sleep?" I asked, while still checking his back and warming his spine under a couple of hot packs.

"I don't sleep very well anymore, I have to get up to pee all the time, and when I get to the toilet, sometimes I just can't."

Another red flag!

"So you try to pee and you can't?" I repeated back to him. "Yeah , that's right. I've been seeing this other chiropractor twice a week for several months now, and nothing has changed. That's why I decided to try someone new."

I asked him when the last time he saw his other chiropractor was and he told me he just saw him last week.

Not good, not good at all.

So, three red flags are enough for me and I said that I couldn't adjust him until he saw his MD. "But I called and they said they couldn't get me in for weeks" he said. "Give me his name," I asked, "I'll call him myself and see what I can do." He signed the medical information release form and I called his doctor. When I got the receptionist on the phone, I told her who I was and that I needed to talk to the doctor personally.

Dr. H. didn't have permission to tell me about Joel, but I had permission to share my findings with him, so I told him, "This guy sounds like he's got some serious prostate problem going on. It's been going on for quite some time now, and his prostate problem has probably traveled into his low back. He is frequently peeing and sometimes peeing blood.

He needs to be seen right away. I would appreciate it if you would book him in as soon as possible." Dr. H. agreed and told the receptionist to get him in as soon as possible. They made him an appointment for later that day and Joel agreed to go.

Joel had let his urinary problem go on for so long that his inflamed prostate, had turned into an enlarged prostate, and his enlarged prostate had become cancerous, and his prostate cancer spread into the nearest bones, which were his sacrum and lumbar spine. The cancer in his spine then referred pain into his low back. His low back had become weakened and misaligned, but that was not the primary problem. The true problem was that our Joel had Prostate cancer, and it had metastasized.

He went for treatment and the doctor said that it would be okay for him to get adjustments, if he wanted to. He felt at this stage, it wouldn't hurt him. So, Joel came back and I adjusted him. He said it made him feel better for a little while, and for that, he was grateful.

The cancer spread throughout his body and Joel became weaker and weaker. In the end he was in a lot of pain. Luckily, a friend had come to stay and care for him during his illness. She brought him to see me once a week and I was happy to do what I could.

In the end, I did go to visit him at his home. On my last visit, he asked me if I would comb his hair. He said he didn't like to look disheveled.

"Of course, I will," I agreed. The last treatment I gave this sweet man was to comb his thinning hair. Not very long after that, Joel passed away.

Regular checkups and routine health screenings are a good way keep an eye on our hidden illnesses. A PSA test would have alerted Joel much sooner to his condition and probably would have saved his life. But, Joel didn't like doctors, so he didn't go. He wouldn't have gone to see Dr. H., that day, if I hadn't made him that appointment, and if I hadn't scared the crap out of him. I scared him because he scared me. I was sure that he had cancer.

All the signs pointed to a severe problem stemming from his long term urinary problem. But, I couldn't say so because aside from the fact that I could very well be wrong, it wasn't my diagnosis to give. The red flags went off like fireworks in my head and alerted me to ask the right questions. I'm sorry he didn't come to see me sooner.

Men over 50 and Black men over 40
(AMA guidelines)
should talk to their doctor about
getting a PSA check
along with their regular check ups.

Chapter 16
Names on my Wall

Ginny comes to see me regularly. She's over 70, but works as hard as a young man. She is constantly pulling her back out because she works too hard, but she loves it. She calls it gardening, and I call it back breaking exertion. Following her bliss, she strains her back, and when she does, she comes to see me. I do the best I can, but it's never easy. She never stretches, she totally overdoes it, and she overdoes it until she can hardly move. Quite often, she'll do something amazingly stupid after she's made an appointment because she knows she's coming to see me and she thinks I can fix her. Every other week, she drags herself into my office and says, "Fix me".

Her usual suspect is a rib right at the level of her heart, just like Roberta, whose rib pain led to gallbladder removal. She has injured that area so many times by either pulling weeds, lifting bags of soil, digging holes, hoeing rows, or yanking hoses that the rib head's attachment to the joint is weak, allowing it to easily twist out of alignment. Her most harmful behavior is yanking hoses, because the combined movement of push, pull, and yank, create the perfect storm, for rib mis-alignments. This rib is on her left side, right over her heart. When it twists out of place, it causes her a stabbing pain, just like a heart attack.

Ginny also has a grown daughter, Marisa. She loves her deeply, but Marisa is off the rails, and Ginny can't fix her. Marissa is not a kid anymore, and has had several bouts with the law, all associated with drug use. The situation with her daughter seems like an obvious association with her recurring heartache and chest pain. Ginny and I have discussed her daughter many times. Her daughter Marissa has entered a difficult path, but at the age of thirty seven, no one can help Marissa to recover, but Marissa. Once again, ribs have names on them and the name on Ginny's painful rib - is Marissa.

I went away on vacation in June to see my new grandchild. I was gone for three weeks. I often ask myself, "If I were to die tomorrow, what would I want to be doing today?" Every time my conclusion is the same, I want to see my grand babies. The kids live in other states too far to drive. So last month, with a glass of wine in one hand, and a credit card in the other, I purchased myself a plane ticket for North Carolina and Oregon. Both are places where my kids live. I closed my office, left a message on my answering machine, and flew off to see my heart's delight.

This last trip in June, while I was gone, Ginny pulled a very long and heavy hose through her garden. She actually had a hose spool pressed against her chest, and cranked and cranked, really hard, using her chest as a brace to stabilize the hose winder. She was already tired before she started, and a tired exhausted body is much easier to injure. She didn't realize it at the time, but that night when she went to sleep, the strained muscles in her chest began to spasm. The rib over her heart twisted, causing pain, and mimicking a heart attack.

She awoke in the middle of the night with excruciating chest pain. She had this pain before, and this familiar pain is usually caused by that pesky rib. She was sure that a massage and adjustment would fix it. She called my office, but I was still in North Carolina. She was feeling desperate and called her friend for help. Her friend, rightfully alarmed, insisted that she go to the emergency room.

Her friend was right to insist, because really, without an immediate adjustment to relieve the pain, and clear up the situation, it appeared to be a heart attack. The pain was on the left side of her chest and traveled down her left arm, and up into her neck. It sounds like a heart attack to me. But in many cases, it's not. Heart attacks in women are difficult to determine. They can hide behind minor signs, such as anxiousness, mild chest pain, pain in the left arm or jaw, pressure or burning in the chest, or even stomach ache. It goes without saying, but if you think your having a heart attack, call your Doctor, or call 911.

Ginny was skeptical of it being a heart attack and was sure it was the same pain she always got, when she overdid it, and just needed a chiropractor. But, with me out of town, unable to adjust her rib and put an end to the episode, her friend insisted that she go to the hospital.

The doctors and nurses were treating it as a heart attack. They did some tests, and after a while, the doctor returned to tell her that the results were inconclusive. They told Ginny that she needed to be admitted overnight for observation and further tests.

She stayed in that mad house, all night, and the next day they finally decided that she didn't have a heart attack. She had probably just strained herself, and could go home now.

I came home a day or two later. Ginny came in right away for her usual adjustment, which relieved her pain. I also recommended that she get a massage to soothe the muscle's in her aching back and chest.

Ginny had muscle strain. It was too bad that the emergency room couldn't tell her that without keeping her over night. They performed an EKG, twice, and did blood tests, checking for the enzymes that would indicate heart damage associated with a heart attack. There were no signs of a heart attack, but they still kept her overnight.

A few weeks later, Ginny received a bill for $60,000. Just getting that bill could have given her a heart attack. Back then, she had no medical insurance because she couldn't afford it. She also couldn't afford a $60,000 dollar medical bill. She'll be paying that darn hospital, $10 dollars a month for the rest of her life.

I have a list of names on my wall. It's a list of people to call in case I intend to leave town for awhile. Ginny's name is at the top.

Heart Attack Signs in Women (American Heart association)

1. Uncomfortable pressure, squeezing, fullness or pain in the center of your chest. It lasts more than a few minutes, or goes away and comes back.
2. Pain or discomfort in one or both arms, the back, neck, jaw or stomach.
3. Shortness of breath with or without chest discomfort.
4. Other signs such as breaking out in a cold sweat, nausea or lightheadedness.
5. As with men, women's most common heart attack symptom, is chest pain or discomfort. But women are somewhat more likely than men to experience some of the other common symptoms, particularly shortness of breath, nausea/vomiting and back or jaw pain.

If you have any of these signs, call 9-1-1 and get to a hospital

Chapter 17
So smart and so stupid

All the local elementary schools have organic gardens, thanks to the vision and perspicacity of Dr. Chris Holden. He sees environmentalism, and children, as our only hope for the survival of our species. You can find him almost every day, out in the garden, with a class of young kids, all digging in the dirt. He teaches them to farm and garden, from the ground up. Just look for the big straw hat that shields his handsome, tanned, face, from the sun.

Most of the children wear similar hats, and they all wear gloves. If you ask them what is their favorite class of the day, and although most children would say recess, these children say garden class. They grow the food and eat what they grow, taking a root or a berry home to show their parents what they've done. They all love Dr. Holden and he loves them too.

Originally born in England, Chris immigrated to Luna thirty years ago. His PHD. is in environmental science and his specialty is in handsome hunk. A few years ago, the local garden club put out a calendar of Luna's most gorgeous bachelors. Chris was featured as Mr. October. The calendar was risque in that all the guys are nude, but like the original calendar girls, the interesting bits are covered somehow. The discreet photo shows his chiseled jaw, his strong back, and his overall flexibility clearly displayed thanks to the yoga pose he holds, while sitting atop a boulder by the side of Luna Lake, in his birthday suit. The calendar made him an instant local celebrity, but even so, his pleasant good nature was not altered, and he is kind and polite to all.

Looking for love should be easy for such a guy, but not for Chris. He was desperately looking for love and companionship, but remained single. He held a position of trust with the school and wouldn't fool around with just anyone. He felt that he needed to set an example of decency, and he did. Attracted to the wild and crazy, although so down to earth himself, was incongruous and difficult. Scores of women flirted with him at the market, or the park, but he wanted what he wanted, and couldn't settle for any less. Chris was looking for love, not convenience.

Young, lovely and talented, Olivia was, and is, a musician. She played music in all the local pubs with some of the best musicians in town. Unbelievably skilled at the saxophone, her jazz skill, and ability to blow that damn horn was amazing. She is definitely a little crazy, but aren't we all?

I remember seeing her at our little town's Earth Day festival. The Solar Winds band was the last band to play for the evening. The moon had come up from behind the mountain and looking up to the stage she was bathed in moonlight from behind, and stood out like a silhouette. Her body bent backward and the sax lifted up from her lips, like Kokopelli with a sax. The sight was magical. The sound was magical. The night was magical. We all fell in love with Olivia that night. It was pretty hard to push Chris's buttons, but when Olivia showed up, she pushed them hard.

The saxophone provided her with food and shelter, but not much else. She was working hard, but hardly getting by. She worked three days a week in the local pub to pay the rent.

One day, Chris walked in while she was mixing drinks and sassing the customers. Flirting wasn't easy for Chris. He was always so serious, and didn't want to look like a Cheshire cat, so he rarely smiled. He almost turned her off with his dour countenance. Luckily she looked past his grim facade, right through to his obvious good looks, great body, clean face and nice clothes, and decided to give him a shot. Lucky for her, and lucky for him.

There was no middle ground. He was madly in love with her, and wanted nothing more than to spend every moment, for the rest of his life, playing house with Olivia.

Chris was working in this country with a green card, so marrying Olivia could earn Chris his citizenship. Although that wasn't his first priority, because any number of women would have been happy to marry Chris. He was, and is, quite a catch. So it was convenient, but not a marriage of convenience. It was obvious to any one, with eyes to see, that Chris and Olivia were lustfully lost in love.

Already a mom, by a previous un-named lover, Olivia came to the marriage complete with a young son, whom Chris took right into his big strong, loving heart.

Everyone loved Olivia. Long silky hair and slim almost boyish figure, man or woman, she musically entered your heart. And that was the truth, man or woman, Olivia was in the game. All that reckless sex, ended with her marriage to Chris. Instantly monogamous, Chris and Olivia seemed finally truly happy. They sealed their union with a beautiful baby girl, whom they both adored. They named her Hope.

Living the eccentric bohemian lifestyle suited Chris just fine. Opening their home to musicians of all kinds, the house was a gathering place for parties and rehearsals. Weekends, they would host all night parties, some lasting for days. What a time that was. I remember attending one event, where we all painted a concrete barrier wall, which extended about sixty feet. We each took a section and painted whatever our artistic eye envisioned. I painted a bluefish chasing its own tail, encircling a big red heart. People would bring food and drinks. Wine and beer was everywhere and the music was amazing. Every weekend was a happening.

But then, the real happening, happened. Olivia uncontrollably attracted to a threesome, was ecstatically rolling around with a couple of people, and neither one of them was Chris. But, of course, Chris walked in, caught them in the act, and was devastated.

The party was over. That's when Chris ended his

relationship with Olivia, and began his relationship with chronic neck pain.

The divorce was painful all around. Although, Olivia really did, and I believe, still does, love Chris, she was unable to control the wild, bohemian, undisciplined, side of herself. All the things that Chris loved about her. He was drawn to the creature that lurked in the shadows, drinking, smoking, playing music, and having sex. What did he expect? When you're attracted to the wild and crazy, you get the wild and crazy. But, seeing her with someone else was more than his heart could take.

Chris was Hope's biological father, but he'd also become a father to Olivia's son, Jeremy. Chris' strong, loving, and hard working nature was just what Jeremy needed. Chris set an example, of a positive male role model that every child needs. When the divorce was finalized, Chris retained partial custody of Hope, and Jeremy as well. The children clung to the stability that Chris had founded for them during the marriage.

Olivia's pain was less obvious, but I'm sure it was there. She was seen about town drowning her pain in the company of local characters. Luna has a lot of those. The sexual parade was colorful and constant. Chris continued to suffer. Seeing her around town with lovers, male and female, young and old was too painful to admit. Rather than make a spectacle of himself, Chris pretended that it didn't bother him. He smiled and shrugged it off. The more he pretended, the worse he felt. Olivia actually looked younger every day. How did she do it? She always had a girlish charm and look about her. She never faded. Must be genetic, or orgasmic. Either way, she got younger and Chris got older.

Unable to move his head, Chris came to see me for massage and chiropractic. He had no idea what he did to cause this problem, but it was effecting his work and his life. He could barely turn his head, and because of it, was actually unsafe on the road. I massaged, heated, and adjusted him. He felt a little better, but I just couldn't alleviate all the pain. I'm usually pretty good at this stuff, but there was something in Chris's neck that was more that bio-mechanical. It was spiritual.

He came to see me again, before he left for his old home in England. He was taking the kids along with him to his childhood home, where the lush countryside and warm hearth could heal their bodies and their souls. They spent the summer chasing Grandpa around the ancient sacred sites of Stonehenge and the surrounding areas. Grandpa was obsessed with ancient places, myths and legends.

When he returned to America, he told me that the whole time that he was in England, he had no pain whatsoever.

So what did that mean? Was he happier in England? Did his stress levels drop, allowing his emotionally charged neck pain to disappear? There was no physical reason that flying in a plane for fourteen hours would make his neck better or that traveling around the world, with two kids would somehow cure his problem, but it did.

As soon as the three of them returned from England, his neck pain came back. He once again, saw Olivia all over town with her new friends. That couldn't have anything to do with anything. Could it? Was he still in love with her, despite her actions? I don't know, but aside from visiting me, Chris got massages and acupuncture from some incredible people here in Luna. Nothing any of us did could make Chris's neck pain go away. Better, but not gone.

The next year Chris went solo to Europe, to once again, help his Dad study Stonehenge. But, this time he would also visit France and Italy. He got as far as France, and met Olivia. Olivia, the second. Guess what? Big surprise! She was crazy! Of course she was, that was his type. Beautiful and crazy. Just like Olivia the first. He was in love, again. And, once again, he fell hard. It was like he lost he ability to reason.

She couldn't come back with him to the states, because she overstayed her visa the last time. She'd been caught and deported, and now she was banished. It took all of his efforts to fight the system and get her re-admitted to the country. First, he had to marry her and she agreed, of course. And then, he had to pay enormous fines. And then, he had to go get her, bring her and all of her stuff here, and then, he had to find a place for her in his house. And then, guess what? He got his pain in the neck back.

When Chris returned, he told me that while he was in Europe, he had no neck pain, at all. He spent a lot of time working with Olivia's situation, so I hadn't seen him for awhile. It took years, money, loads of paperwork and tireless fortitude to get Olivia the second back into the country and living in Luna. Now that he and Olivia the second were living in his house, everything should have been fine, but it wasn't. His neck pain was gone while he worked in England and vacationed in France. But now that he was back on Luna soil, married, and living with Olivia in the states, his pain was back and doubled.

French, exotic, tiny, lithe and lovely, Olivia the second, seemed just as bohemian as Olivia the first, but not as talented and not as cool. When I first met her she seemed aloof, cold and calculating. She dressed in scarves, and not just around her neck. Her dresses actually looked like they were made of scarves, all wispy, ethereal and artsy.

Friends and family laughed, "Olivia the Second!"

"No, no, just Olivia." insisted Chris. But, the joke had started and we all loved a good laugh.

Temperamental and selfish, with a flair for the dramatic and regal, she began to spend his money and dominate his home.

Once again, he came to my office regularly,

suffering from severe neck pain. He professed happiness, but his demeanor and physical appearance told me otherwise. Seeing him so often, it was clear to us both, that something was wrong.

One day, after hot packs and massage, he confessed his abject depression. "I'm not happy. I don't know what to do. I tried so hard to get her here and now that she's here, I'm miserable. I must be crazy."

"No", I said, "you were crazy to jump head first into this crazy project to get her into the country. You were so caught up in the struggle to succeed, you didn't notice that it was the challenge that had you hooked. You probably should have taken a little more time to actually get to know her."

Trapped in his nightmare he was no longer seen around town with Olivia the Second. He was miserable, and didn't know what to do. When it came to crazy women, Chris was helpless. She had her teeth into him like a badger.

Hope and Jeremy, a little more grown now, advised him to get divorced and stay single. Jeremy was almost eighteen and nobody's fool. He could see Chris's blind spot, and begged him to divorce Olivia the Second. He also suggested that afterward, if he wanted, he and Chris could move in together. He was working and wanted his own place, but sharing a space with Chris would be amazing, and helpful to them both.

Olivia, the First, was still in his life because Chris is a nice guy. He loves the kids, and she is their mother. But, between separating from Olivia the Second, and watching Olivia the First, flirt with men all over town, he was close to a nervous breakdown. Instead of a nervous breakdown, he had a neck breakdown. Being a door mat for two crazy women was making Chris more and more downtrodden. I mentioned to him that all his work with the huge, rock boundaries of Stonehenge, hadn't done his own boundaries any good.

"You've got to stop being a snot rag, Chris. Learn patience, and erect some boundaries around your personal space, and around your heart. You can be attracted to someone without immediately marrying them. Get to know them a little better first. It's the wise thing to do. Cut your losses and move on."

No matter what I did, his neck never released. We tried everything, and every time he came, we spoke about his impossible situation. I wasn't alone in my feeling about Olivia the Second, most of his friends disliked her immensely, and were sure she had used him to overcome her immigration status.

Olivia, the Second, wasn't going down without a fight. She spread rumors all over town that Chris had taken advantage of her and had brought her here under false pretenses.

Chris was horrified that his friends and neighbors would all think he was a jerk. He begged her to stop slandering him, trying to appeal to her decency.

Confused, but searching for enlightenment, he

retreated to Jeremy's house. With his step-son for support, he succeeded in obtaining his divorce, but not his freedom. At no time during this process did his neck ever recover.

Even after the divorce, Olivia the Second continued to spread vicious lies and tell ridiculous stories of Chris' cruel treatment of her. Anyone who knew Chris, knew they weren't true, and that's what I told him. "No one who knows you, believes her." I said. "You have to let go of what she and her angry friends think of you. What other people think of you is none of your business. What you know to be true is all that matters. You can't please everyone all of the time. No one can."

Chris began to run into Olivia the Second wherever he went. Whenever he went to his usual environmental meetings or the trivia night at the local pub, she would be there, sitting at the table by the door. All the places that Chris could would frequent --- Surprise! There she was.

"Isn't that a coincidence?" he said to me. "No, Chris." I said, " It's not. She's stalking you, you idiot."

"Do you really think so?" he said.

"Yes, Yes! I think so, I know so. You're so smart and so stupid. Don't play the game with her. Don't let her goad you into anger or remorse. Pretend that you don't see her and let her go. Don't answer her calls, her texts, her e-mails, or her demands. Cut her off."

Weeks passed. Then one afternoon, when he had come for his usual appointment, after the usual, heat and massage, one more time, I gently attempted to adjust his neck.

It was the crack heard round' the world! The noise was deafening. In shock and elation I stood stunned at the head of the table. We were both shocked and astonished. The breakthrough, that we had both been waiting for, had occurred. The spell was broken. He had taken a step up to freedom. Not only was he free from the Olivias, free from trying to please everyone but himself.

He's still out there searching for a crazy girl, who won't break his heart. He hasn't given up hope, but he's grown from the pain. He's back to visiting Stonehenge every summer, perhaps he'll fall in love with a wispy druid. **And perhaps**, he'll take the time to get to know her better.

He has learned to love himself and he doesn't need to prove his worth to anyone. I don't know what finally opened his eyes. But he is living with his stepson, and best friend, and he's dating a wider range of lovely, crazies. He's open to minor league crazy, instead of going straight for the major league, home run hitter, kind of crazy.

His neck is better. I didn't do anything different that day than I usually do. When the time was right, his neck released, and popped like a champagne cork.

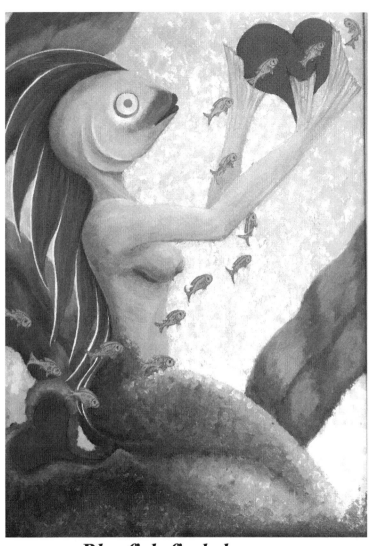

Bluefish finds love

Chapter 18
Put what? Where?

Lovely, wealthy, and in constant pain, Carla was in the unfortunate position of needing some one to put their finger up her butt. Well known for her singing and songwriting capabilities, one night after singing at a club, she'd fallen off a bar stool, straight down onto her butt. Ever since her fall, her butt pain was killing her and she couldn't sit down without pain, or a pillow. Her doctor and his x-rays told her that her bones weren't broken, but she was left with coccodynia (pain in the coccyx), which is the medical term for a pain in the butt.

At the base of the spine and forming the posterior portion of the pelvic bowl, is the sacrum. Just below the sacrum looking like a vestigial tiny tail is the coccyx. Sometimes, as a result of falling on your butt, straight down onto a hard surface, your coccyx becomes subluxated. If it doesn't reposition itself back to its proper place, your butt hurts forever.

As a chiropractor I can adjust the coccyx, but, you guessed it, I have to do it by putting my finger up the patients butt, up to the level of the coccyx and then gently tug the coccyx back into position. Nobody wants to have that done, but that's what it takes, and quite a few people have benefited by this chiropractic adjustment. Luckily for them, my hand and my fingers are small. Plus, I'm a woman, a mother, and a grandmother. These last two job titles have put me in contact with wiping and attending to babies butts of all sexes and I am not weird about it.

I never adjust a coccyx on the first visit. I advise the patient that such a procedure could be necessary if whatever we do today doesn't make the pain go away. Thereby giving them the option of never coming back. But, if a sacral or pelvic adjustment doesn't do the trick, they come back for the coccyx adjustment because they are, by that time, desperate. It's not a comfortable adjustment, but it works. I sent Carla home to think about it and she came back in a few days saying "Please, just do it!" The actual movement is almost undetectable, but the effect is remarkable.

Immediately after the adjustment, she was relieved and grateful. This particular adjustment is usually a one shot deal. It doesn't need to be done more than once, unless, of course, you fall on your butt again. Happy not to return, I see her around town all the time. I ask her how she is doing and she always says, "I'm doing Great". I know what she means, she means her butt feels fine, thank you very much, and we don't mention the details.

The medical community has no cure for most cases of Coccodynia, other than, rest, use a donut pillow, and try cortisone injections.

If you have a pain in the butt and you think you can trace it back to a fall, go see your chiropractor.

Segments of the spinal column

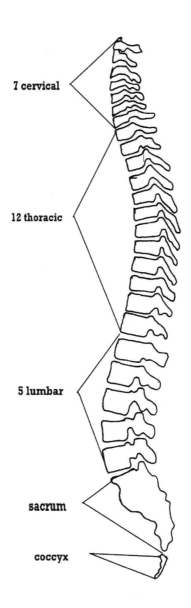

7 cervical

12 thoracic

5 lumbar

sacrum

coccyx

Chapter 19
When did I get so old?

I may be in my sixties, but I still feel like I'm 21.

As I get older, I lay in my bed at night and say to myself "How did I get here?"

I may be thirty, forty, fifty, or sixty, but I still feel like I'm 21. I look back over my life and try to find the moment that I became older. It all happened so slowly that I just didn't notice the turning of the wheel. Exercise and Yoga keeps me limber, but I get tired more easily, and I just can't do some of the things that I used to do, and I'm wise not to try.

If I ever decide to go skiing again, I'll have to get back into skiing shape, starting slowly and building up to my old level of expertise. Guarding against the horrific torn ligament or broken bone. I can't just show up at the slope, with the rest of the young squirts, and those who have regularly kept up with their skiing, and go right up to the double diamond. That would be stupid!

I often make this comparison when I talk to my clients about going back to the gym after many years of inactivity and body neglect. You can't just go back to the same levels that you were at twenty years ago. Even being away from your normal fitness regime for a few weeks, can leave you weaker and less toned. You need to cut back on your workout level, allowing yourself to build up to your old abilities,

OR you can easily hurt yourself.

Sometimes, when older guys go to the gym, they see other guys in so much better shape than they are. In an effort to compete, or thinking they can regain their youthful vigor, they over work and over do. That's the worst, it usually doesn't end well.

Guys are just as much, or more, conscious of their physique, in a gym, as women are. With or without the fancy work out clothes, guys just want to look good and feel young.

Men strive to be virile and strong, and they often think of themselves as they were in their high school years, as though it was yesterday. Even into their fifties, men remember playing sports and think they're still in the same youthful shape.

I've heard fifty year old men tell me that they play football. Looking at them, they don't look like they play football. When I ask them, when was the last time they played, they tell me proudly, "In high school." It's been thirty years since they've been in high school, but they still, puff out their chest, suck in their stomach, and say "I play football."

It's magical thinking, I guess, like lying bed and feeling like I'm 21, but the fantasy can set us up for a rude reality check. Both men and women, will attempt to do something that was no problem when they were in high school, but is foolish to try in their current state of fitness, twenty, thirty, or forty years later.

My friend, Dave, has always kept himself in

really good shape, but faced with the passage of time, he has recently begun to compete with men thirty years younger. He actually believes that he can easily keep up.

As we age, we don't heal as quickly as we used to. We can still maintain excellent health, but we need to supplement our high quality, diet with extra vitamins, minerals, and essential fatty acids, and engage in a regular exercise program without over doing it. A good trainer is a great way to workout without getting on the wrong track.

After several weeks of competing with a much younger group of guys at the gym, Dave threw out his shoulder. He came to me for help, but wouldn't listen when I told him to take it easy and allow it to heal. I could adjust his shoulder and spine, but I couldn't adjust his thinking.

He shouldn't have returned to his regime full bore, but he did anyway. Then his neck tweaked and then, finally, his low back twisted. Angry and in pain he returned to my office for me to 'fix him,' but I couldn't, and I told him so. I told him that none of your injuries are healing because you don't give yourself time to heal. Lay off your work out for a while. Go see your Doctor. Talk to your Trainer. Take time to recuperate.

"NO," he said, "I do feel a little better now, and I can heal while I train. I've always been able to bounce back, no matter what."

"But, you're not bouncing back" I said, "you're

falling apart! You're not a kid anymore!"

Dave got really pissed off at that last remark and left my office in a huff. He wound up going to an orthopedic surgeon who told him that he had a torn rotator cuff in his shoulder. He was angry that his body had let him down. But really, he'd let his body down. By not appreciating its need for care, repair and convalescence, he beat his poor old body to a pulp.

He underwent rotator cuff surgery and was never the same. They told him it would take six weeks and he would be back to normal, but six months later, he was still pretty stiff and sore. He doesn't even go to the gym anymore because he's angry, depressed, in pain, and in denial.

My handsome friend, Dave, went from one extreme to another, fanatically overdoing his work out, and then stopping completely. He would have been so much better off working at a steady pace, balancing his muscle building with his stretching routines.

All of Dave's injuries could have been avoided by using a trainer and listening to them. Or at least, listening to me and using bodywork, chiropractic and holistic remedies to speed his healing. He needed to cut back on his overzealous workout regimen and allow himself time for recuperation. Adding healing herbs and life extending supplements can help with speedy recovery and youthful vigor. One herb that I heartily recommend as a whole body tonic is

Echinacea, in tablet or tincture, it helps every system in your body.

I've always liked Dave, and most women found him attractive, but that wasn't enough for Dave. He pushed himself to the point of injury, and beyond, and that's a recipe for disaster.

When embarking on an exercise and fitness routine,
start slowing and work within your limits.

Always balance your workouts with stretching.

Echinacea every day enhances feelings of well being
and supports healthy aging.

Chapter 20
Emotions can kill you

"Cancer" that was all I heard. Everything the doctor said after that, he may as well have been talking to himself, because I didn't hear a thing.

"Cancer, I have cancer and I don't understand why. I'm so damn healthy!" I thought to myself. I'm strong, and tough, and smart, and miserable. Yes, if I'm honest, I was miserable. Miserable in my marriage, which I was determined to keep together at all costs, even if it costs me my life.

I always imagined that I would be a better mother than the mother that I had. That I would be happier and more loving, and that my life would be like the lives of the people I'd seen on TV, Ozzie and Harriet, Donna Reed and Dr. Stone, June and Ward Cleaver. (If your under 50, you may not recognize these names, all from the black and white TV. sit-coms of my youth.) They made it look so easy, but I had no idea how hard it would be to achieve.

I was determined to make my marriage work. Striving for such an unrealistic model is the essence of overwhelming stress. I have always been so proud of my determination, but now, my determination was leading me down a path to disaster.

I discovered that there is a personality type for cervical cancer. Today they call the study, psycho-oncology. Back then it wasn't recognized.   After researching the situation, I could see the common personality traits in myself, which are: Number one- Taking on the responsibility to make everyone happy, Number two: Saying Yes when you really want to say No. Number three- Doing more and more for everyone else at the sacrifice of your self, and Number four- Being a human doormat. All these activities, lead to so much stress that your body can't cope with it anymore and then, it starts to affect your heart, your soul, and your immune system.

Overwhelming stress puts such a burden on your adrenal glands and your entire endocrine system that every hormone producing organ in your body gets thrown off kilter. It's all associated with the hypothalamic, pituitary, adrenal axis, (the HPA axis). This glandular triangle is what mediates the stress cycle and the function of the immune system. When you're over stressed, the excess cortisol that you produce, throws off the balance between your mid brain, (hypothalamus, and pituitary glands) and the adrenal gland. When this happens, you can gain weight, get indigestion, have irritable bowel syndrome, chronic fatigue syndrome, high blood pressure, diabetes, or even psychological problems of depression and worse.

When your HPA axis is out of balance, your body's an open door for invading cancer cells to take over. Your soldiers at the gate are too tired and exhausted to notice that the enemy has landed. There are supplements and exercises that will help, but at the time, I hadn't started on my path to chiropractic college and I didn't know enough about natural remedies and holistic health to save my own life.

That horrible day, after leaving the Doctors office, I couldn't go home. I was devastated and I didn't want to upset the family with my death sentence. Another nail to my own coffin, keeping it all inside and not sharing. But, I did have one special friend, that I could share with, she lived in the orange orchard at the east end of town. I headed that way like a blind person in a storm. I broke down crying almost as soon as I got there.

I walked out into the rows of blossoming orange trees, and sank to the ground. Tears filled my eyes, until I couldn't see anymore, and slowly I began to lift from the ground. I was leaving my body behind as my super conscious was starting to float out above the trees, into the blue sky and beyond. My grief had taken me out of my body, and into the higher realms of being. God was showing me the workings of the universe.

The air was filled with bright white lines, like laser beams cutting through space. It was like lace work and where the threads intersected the nodes shone like stars, glowing brighter with the increased energy of union. I could see and understand, how every molecule effected another. We are not separate and apart, we are inextricable tied to all things, all the threads connected to make a beautiful intricate pattern. If a stitch is dropped the whole cloth is changed, and every corner is affected. Like granny's beautiful exquisite doily made of stardust.

Looking down I could see my life's path. I wondered, how did I get here? I could see the dotted line leading me on a wild ride, to the place in the trees, where I sat that day. My whole life played before me like reruns of "I Love Lucy." I never meant for it to be this way. Yes, I wanted children and a family, but I wanted it to be a happy life, not so hard all the time. Looking back, I realize that it all came down to me. Not that I needed to do more, but I needed to do more for me, and cut back on the expectations that I had for myself. I was trying too hard. I was worn out all the time and everyone suffered, my beloved children, my husband and most of all, ME.

So, I thought about my life and realized, that somehow, I had made the choices that had brought me to that spot. I could continue on with my life in that way, and probably die of the disease, or I could change my life. I could turn everything upside down. I wasn't happy in my marriage, but I took a sacred oath to ride it out. I swore to god, till death do us part. On the horns of a dilemma, I had to choose to pull the rug out from under all the loved ones in my universe, or die.

At the same time that I was facing this life crisis, my girlfriend, Sherry, who lived around the corner and had three children, coincidentally, all very close to the ages of my three children. Was having a crisis of her own.

Her family seemed so very happy and her husband was a handsome, hardworking, sweetheart. She was a bouncy, heavy set girl with rosy cheeks. A child at heart, one of her favorite things to do, was to take one of her three girls out of school and sneak away to the amusement park for the day.

Dear Sherry was pregnant again, she said that she, her husband and the three kids were thrilled. Being pregnant can be a challenge, even when you're thrilled. Sherry had morning sickness, really bad, every morning. She was throwing up a lot. So much so that she was weak and dehydrated. One morning, after finding her on the floor of the bathroom, her husband decided to take her the hospital.

Throwing up every morning depletes you of your fluids. Sherry had fainted from dehydration. First thing that the doctors decided to do, was to put a catheter in her and give her some fluids. She was so dehydrated it was difficult for the nurse to find a vein in her arm. She tried several times and then decided to put the catheter into a vein in her chest. I don't know why, and I'm not sure that it was a good idea, because somehow, Sherry blew an embolism that went to her brain. Her last words were, "I feel funny" and then she died.

The local hospital was in a panic. Her husband was white and numb, from the shock. She was to be held for autopsy, but instead they shipped her immediately to the mortuary for embalming. Shortly thereafter the attending nurse disappeared. And then, the hospital lost her bed records. Even if no one had done anything wrong, it sure looked like the hospital was trying to cover something up.

Long story short, the judge decided that a fairly healthy young woman went into the hospital that morning, for routine nursing care, and a dead one came out. The hospital was held responsible, they were ordered to give money for her three young daughters in a trust for their future. But, of course, that wouldn't replace their mother or mend their broken hearts, nor would it help their father to cope with the loss, of the love of his life.

After the diagnosis of cancer was given to me, two days earlier, I was blindly going through the motions of my life, when I heard the news of Sherry. I remember sitting on my bed, and thinking, I could cling desperately to my unhappy marriage, trying to keep my family together, killing myself with cancer, or I could change my life completely.

Before my diagnosis of cancer, my biggest concern was that my children would come from a broken home. After what had happened to Sherry, I saw the alternative, I could die and my children could be motherless, just like Sherry's were now. I took the events as a sign from God. He was telling me it was "OK" to break my oath. I chose to utterly and completely change my life. Turn it upside down, and the entire family along with it.

I tried to talk to my husband, but he was

belligerent and stubborn, big surprise. He didn't want to see that we had a problem. He's a Taurus, and they have a reputation for being stubborn. I finally convinced him to go to counseling with me. The young intern that we saw, told us, that because of my history of childhood abuse, he wouldn't be able to help us as a couple, unless I went for personal counseling on my own. The verdict of the inexperienced counselor offered a clear avenue for my husband to blame me for everything, and take the stand that I was the one that needed the help, not him. Feeling vindicated of any responsibility for the problems of our marriage, he refused to go for counseling or therapy of any kind, anymore.

I decided to go on alone. I found a wonderful counselor who showed me clearly, I could be and do anything I wanted. Life was limitless. All I had to do was make up my mind to do something, and then, just do it!

With the picture of Sherry's motherless children clearly in my mind, I filed for divorce from my husband, grieving the whole time for what I was doing. I was in pain and torment over my decision, but I knew that I had to do it, in order to live. My children were in tears and in pain. They have never forgiven me for destroying the family. I don't know how he could have been so blind, but my husband was in shock too. He never thought I would go through with my threat, although I warned him many times. "I swear to god, if something doesn't change I'm gonna get a divorce." All he said was "go ahead."

Nobody knew that god had talked to me personally. On my knees in prayer, he had given me permission to choose a different path. I went to therapy for seven years. I had several different therapists, some good, and some not so good. But, they all helped me along my way. I knew that I had to change my life. I couldn't turn everyone else's life upside down and not turn my own life upside down as well. There had to be a purpose to all this pain.

My life now, is very different from what it was. I'm stronger. I no longer look to other people for my happiness, or my living. In order to properly support myself and my children, I went back to school. At thirty six years old, I entered chiropractic school. After four grueling hard years, after which, I received the clinic proficiency scholarship award, and graduated at the top of my class.

I started to work while I was still in school. I practiced on everything and everyone, my kids, my friends, my dogs, everyone. I drove them crazy, taking care of them, but I take care of everyone I meet, that's who I am, and that's what I do. But, it's also what a mom does. But now, I take care of myself too. I no longer give up me, to help others. I can listen and not feel the need to interfere, for a healer that's a big deal, but we all must have boundaries.

During this transformation, I went in for surgery to have my cancerous cells removed. I decided against Chemo and radiation. I'm not saying that I recommend that for everyone, I'm just saying that it was right for me. I knew that once I broke free from my turmoil, I would be alright again. I knew that if I could change my life, I could change my health, and thereby change my destiny. By claiming my strength and embracing the female warrior within me, I could survive it all.

It's a funny thing about life, when you have a character challenge at one stage in your life, you will have it again at another level. If you passed the first test, then the next encounter with the challenge will be at a higher level. My choices at that time, have led me here. I am at a higher level of challenge than I was back then. I do have regrets. I sometimes think that I may have failed the last test because I'm not sure if I'm at a higher level, or at the same place all over again.

Forging ahead, I know that I'm doing pretty well, because I'm happy almost all the time. So that's a good measure of success. Now, I recognize the personality profile of cancer candidate. When I see an overworked, exhausted, unappreciated person, unable to say no, unable to step back and relax, putting themselves last, unhappy and miserable with a perpetual smile on their face, I recognize it right away. Whether or not I say something, is a choice I make at the time, but I know it, when I see it. Not everyone with these traits will become cancer patients, but the situation leads to immune exhaustion and sickness of some sort.

My friend, Dot, has cancer now. She called me the other day from her parent's house, where she was visiting. She has the same type of cancer that I had. I told her that I would be there for her, but I also told her that if she wanted to live, she was going to have to examine her life, involve herself with Psychotherapy, and be willing to change.

I recommend Echinacea, Withania, and Licorice root, as whole food adrenal supports. Every day take total body vitamin, mineral and essential fatty acid supplements. See your chiropractor for adjustments. Completely eliminate sugar, high fructose corn syrup and processed food from the diet. Practice Yoga and meditation. All these practices to help support a properly functioning hypothalamic- pituitary-adrenal axis.

Sometimes life taps us on the shoulder and sometimes life pulls the rug out from under us. We must pay attention to what we tell ourselves, consciously or unconsciously, because obviously, our emotions can kill us.

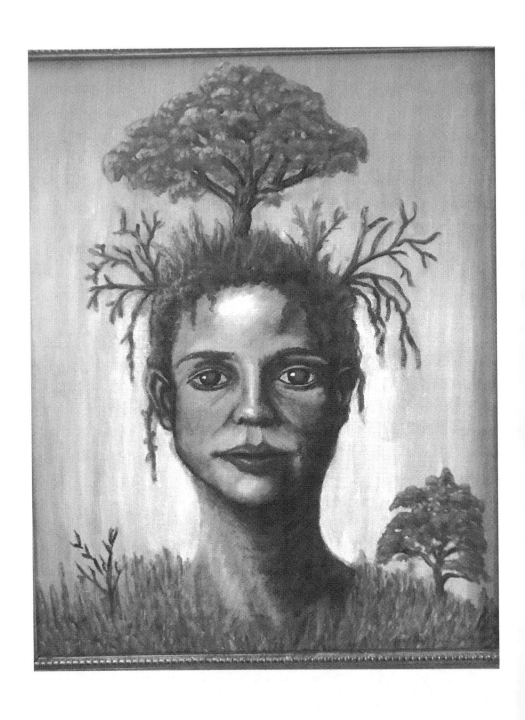

Earth energy shoots up out of my head

Chapter 21
The Chiropractor sandwich

Russell changed his name to Rusty Bullet. The name fit him to a Tee. He was six foot six, of red haired, Viking, mountain man, crossed with a Renaissance man. Poet, architect, sculptor, masseuse, and yes, four hundred pounds, all my patient. At that weight, he is more that three times my size. But, I am always up to the task. I have gymnastic rings that hang from my ceiling. I use the rings to balance myself when I walk on people. A friend of mine put them in for me because I've always been short and small, and using my feet, is sometimes easier, than using my hands. As a child, I used my feet to walk on my brothers back, to make him feel better.

Rusty seemed like a happy, jolly man, but that could be, because he was always stoned. Remember the Cancer profile? He smoked pot constantly to cover his overwhelming unhappiness. Rusty was an orphan, and had been looking, all his life, for his father, who was obviously a Viking, because there is no mistaking Rusty for anything other than a Viking. He thought for a while that his dad was the wrestling star "The Undertaker", but he couldn't get in contact with the man to find out. They did look remarkably similar, in face and physique. If the undertaker was anything like Rusty he probably had a bunch of woman gushing all over him.

Women loved Rusty. He wasn't just big and handsome, but also a warm and loving gentle giant. The combination had the women swooning.

Unfortunately, but not surprising, his obesity was causing problems for his back, knees, legs and worst of all, his heart. I counseled him constantly about diet and exercise and he would smile and promise compliance. But, the next time I saw him, it was obvious that he had not been, in the least bit, compliant.

Whenever he came in for an adjustment, he would joke about me walking on his back, dressed in a black leather cat suit (like Catwoman). I thought it was a riot, and we laughed about it every time he came in. We both had fun imagining me in that cat suit. Perhaps I can find one to wear to the next masquerade party. I'll make sure to post the picture on my website.

One day, he brought his lovely wife in to see me. She had been having back pain for awhile. At first, I thought it may have something to do with emotional pain because it was centered right behind her heart. It might have been emotional, when the problem first started, but that was a while ago. She had been ignoring it, for maybe, too long.

She led a rich spiritual life and had recently undergone a vision quest. She was sure that the grueling ordeal, of fasting for days, alone, in the woods, had caused her back problem. But, when questioned, she was uncertain, if the pain started before, or after, her trial in the mountains.

She had put off seeing me, or anyone else, for fear of the worst. After examining her, I feared the worst as well, and sent her immediately to an MD.

"You're frightening me," she said.

"You're frightening me too," I said. So off she went, pissed off that I had made such a big deal of it all.

She was very shortly diagnosed with a cancer that had reached her pericardium. She quickly began to weaken. They began treatments. When I saw her again, she had lost her hair and was wearing a cowboy bandana on her bald head.

As we stood on the sidewalk, in front of the coffee shop, she thanked me for my help, and she asked me if she was going to be okay. A question for which I am not qualified to answer. I warmly assured her, that anything was possible with truth, enlightenment, and love. It's up to you, Sara, not me. Radiation and chemo were bombarding her cancerous cells, but it was all too late and much too quickly, she died.

Rusty was devastated and his already crappy health, declined further, along with his happy, jolly attitude. He continued to sculpt and smoke pot, but he never recovered from the loss.

Smoking pot has the inherent side effect of giving people the munchies. Losing weight while getting stoned is almost impossible. With his weight ballooning, his knees couldn't hold him up any longer. His only comfort was being in the pool. The buoyancy took the immense weight of his poor, aching, joints. Getting into the pool was easy, getting out became harder and harder.

He came in to see me, many moons later, and he was bigger than ever. I used to be able to get my arms around him to adjust his mid back. If I could just get my arms around him, I could adjust him. As big as he had become, I couldn't do that any longer. I could still hang from the ceiling and adjust him with my feet. But, that doesn't work for everything, and adjusting him was becoming almost impossible.

What I could do was helping, so he sill wanted me to work on him. One day he called for an appointment, his back was hurting him again, along with his broken heart. Some of Sara's old boyfriends were out visiting, attending her memorial. When Rusty came in for his treatment, he brought them along with him. I had seen both of these guys before, as patients, in my office, so we were all old friends.

I was having such a hard time trying to adjust Rusty that I asked the guys if they could help me. I thought that if I wrap my arms around Rusty, as best I could, then one of these big guys could get on top of us, and when I gave the signal, he could drop his body weight down onto the two of us. I was hoping that the combined poundage would be enough force to move the bones. He would be the brawn and I would be the finesse. They were both over six feet tall and quite handsome. The one guy, Chris, had actually been a very close and intimate friend of Sara.

First, I wrapped my arms around Rusty. And then, Kevin, the other gorgeously handsome guy, wrapped his arms around me. Thinking that this was going to be amazing, I gave the signal, and Kevin dropped his two hundred and twenty pounds, like a ton of bricks, right down on top of me.

Well, I wasn't actually the finesse, I was more like the cream cheese. I was compressed between the two of them like a squashed sandwich. But, the whole crazy thing worked. We managed to adjust that spot on Rusty's back, where the pain was stabbing him, right into his heart.

Chris sat on the stool, in the corner, and laughed hysterically the whole time. We were all laughing like crazy, once I got my breath back.

I'm short and small, so when it comes to working with big people, I have to be extremely creative, and resilient. Kevin and Rusty were tall, strong, and handsome. With me in the middle, we made a chiropractor sandwich. I don't mind being the cheese, when these two gorgeous hunks are the bread. Sorry, no pictures of this. I wish I had one to include with this story, like they say, it would have been "one for the book".

I found out later, that Chris, had been Sara's lover. She was married and in love with Rusty, but for a very long time, she had also been in love with Chris. Her divided feelings could have been causing her heartache, tension, and stress, setting her up for heart disease and Cancer. Most of what I know about her, I learned after she died, so It's really hard for me, to even guess what caused her heart to weaken.

At the memorial, we all found out, that Sara had privately owned some land in Colorado. She left the property, not to Rusty, but to Chris.

That was an unexpected surprise for everyone, including Rusty.

Rusty was broken and lost without Sara, his wife of twenty five years. Living in a fog of pot smoke, he began the drudgery of living in the house without her. For the past three months, while she was sick, the house had been full of nurses, caregivers, and friends. Francesca, Sara's lovely french nurse, who cared for Sara during her last days, stayed on in the house after Sara passed, and helped keep things going.

About a week after Sara died, Francesca told Rusty that Sara had visited her in a dream, and spoke to her. Sara, in the dream, told Francesca, that Rusty was lonely and needed love. Francesca was supposed to take care of Rusty for her. In other words, take Sara's place as Rusty's wife.

Pleasantly surprised at this turn of events during his time of grief, Rusty agreed to give it a try, and the two set up housekeeping together. Whatever money Rusty had, Francesca found a way to spend. Rusty was distracted from his grief by the amazing, full bodied, attention that he was getting from Francesca.

But, the attention came at a price and Francesca didn't come cheap. She bought whatever she wanted, clothes, CD's, jewelry, even a very expensive Maltese puppy. After several months, Rusty was broke, and Francesca was gone, along with her pirate booty and the puppy.

The grieving process that had been postponed, due to all the shenanigans, fell upon him with a vengeance. Not long after his beloved wife died, and the French nurse drove him to poverty, Rusty fell into a pit of pot smoke and junk food. Sinking deeper and deeper into depression, and gaining pounds over pounds, his heart could no longer stand the strain, and Rusty, passed away.

I've had many experiences with patients taking a turn for the worse when a loved one dies. Like Claudine, who kept her dead brother alive in her chest, and was not willing to let him go.

In spite of the swinging lifestyle, Sara and Rusty were soul mates, and both died from the broken heart of lost love.

Takotsubo syndrome strikes again.

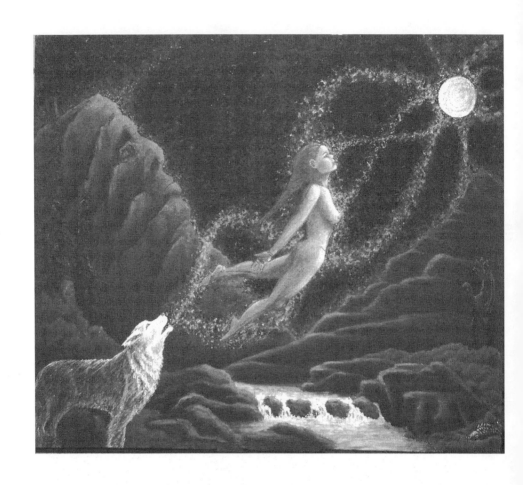

Transcendence

**Traveling to the power of the full moon,
on the howl of a wolf**

Chapter 22
My personal bubble

Floating through the crowd like a diaphanous ghost, Maureen glowed with the flame of true beauty and grace. Like a modern day Grace Kelly, (Princess of Monaco), she charmed the men, and then, laughed with the ladies, about the men.

She knew who was who, and she knew how to pretend like it didn't matter. A gorgeous carnival huckster, she was a barker for charities and good causes. She was the finest, most glamorous fund raiser around. She had all the right connections with all the beautiful people and the beautiful people wannabes. The wannabes sometimes gave her more money than the be's. It was all for good causes and charities. Some people just know how to do that stuff, and Maureen knew how. It was her super power.

As she flitted about the room, I noticed that she seemed to connect with everyone, yet connect with no one. She stopped by my table to give me a hug and say hello, smelling like springtime in the Rockies, and looking like an angel.

"I need to come see you", she said, "my neck is killing me." And then like a butterfly, she was gone.

"I'm getting another headache, and I feel nauseous." she whispered, when she arrived for her appointment. She had secret aches and pains, because no one was supposed to know that she wasn't perfect. Like bird in the wild, as long as you look healthy, you're fine. She made a point of always looking beautiful, vital, and well dressed.

Her handsome husband was rich and talented. Her fabulously elegant home, was at the top of the tallest mountain around, a few miles outside of town. I loved that place, and it had the most amazing views. It's crazy, but If you sat on the toilet in her upstairs bathroom, you could see the ocean from one window, and the mountains from the other. It's my favorite bathroom ever. I once saw a doe and her fawn, grazing calmly in the grass, while I was sitting in that exact spot.

I loved her house, but I hated the rugged, narrow and treacherous road that led up to it. I'm always afraid of the blind curves. The speed limit was ten miles per hour, but I had seen people come barreling down that mountain, like it was a raceway.

One evening, shortly after one of her fantastic events, while she was on her way home, she met another driver, coming around the blind curve like a runaway train. It hit her car head on, slamming into her small car and crunching it like an accordion. Everyone died, except Maureen. Hanging on, by a thread and a prayer, she collapsed against the crumpled metal and began to bleed to death.

Her neighbor, Marshall, and his pup, Asta, were having an evening stroll when the accident took place. Marshall was close enough to see the whole horrible thing and he immediately called for help. Talking to the dispatcher, he approached Maureen's car. When he saw the wound that opened up to her skull, his gut twisted.

Unbelievably, she was still conscious and moaning. Getting closer, he could hear her speaking. Like a zombie movie, looking dead, but still alive, through the blood and torn flesh, she spoke. Trying to comfort her through the jagged glass of the smashed window, Marshall repeated over and over again, that everything would be okay. Sitting with her for almost an hour, he gently touched her hand and told her to hold on, help was coming!

Her skull was smashed and blood was everywhere. Her body was trapped and her shoulder, knee, ankle, and several ribs were broken.

The driver of the other car had no insurance. The hospital costs drained her personal insurance and finances, until there was nothing left. Years of raising money for other people, opened the door for other people to raise money for her. She had become a charitable cause. The concert in the park raised more than anyone expected, but it was still not enough to cover all the bills. However, the love and support she received, helped almost as much as the money.

Years later, she is still deaf in one ear, crippled in one leg, frozen in one wrist and in constant facial, neck and head pain.

She limped into my office, leaning on her cane. I

was shocked to see this once beautiful woman, struggling for posture and presence.

I wanted so much to help her. I tried everything I could think of. If I could turn back time, I would have gladly done it. I called for the energies of the universe to shine down and have mercy on her. Taking it personally, I prayed for guidance, strength and knowledge. I studied obscure body work techniques, hoping to find something, to help free her from the constant pain.

In my free time, I constructed a custom, thermal face wrap, filled with lavender, to warm in the microwave and lay across her face, trying to soothe her pain. I was constantly on the lookout for new techniques or tools that might help her. I became obsessed with finding a way to relieve her suffering. It broke my heart to see her like that. She said my treatments helped, but she was still in so much pain. I wasn't satisfied, and ached to do more.

She became a part of my prayers, and I fell asleep one night, while mentally searching for therapeutic cures. If you ask the universe for help before you go to sleep, sometimes the answer pops into your head when you wake up.

The next morning, I awoke, not with my prayed for answer, but paralyzed and in pain. My face hurt, my ear hurt, everything hurt. When I tried to get up, I had trouble walking. Terrified, I sank to the floor. Searching for answers. Laying there in a lump, wracked with pain, I had an epiphany. I had done the one thing that body workers must never do, I over empathized and left myself unguarded.

In my desire to help, I had crossed the line, and I allowed our energies to coalesce. I had absorbed her painful energy. Like Claudine had done with her brother, I took on Maureen's pains and problems.

In shock and disbelief, I had no idea what to do next. I clearly saw the connection between Maureen's pain and my own. I had heard about this kind of thing happening, but it had never happened to me before. I had to cancel my patients for the day. I called a friend who's a world class, mind-body worker, and massage therapist. He came to my house and brought his table. I remember being crumpled and devastated, on the floor crying. He massaged my neck and head, while talking to me about the boundaries that we must maintain, when we work with people. My youngest son was home at the time, the poor thing was just as terrified as I was.

Gently speaking, to me and my son, Gerry explained to us both, about human energy fields, auras, and the healing field. Keeping a boundary between ourselves and other people was the only way to keep from taking on negative energy. Whether the energy is painful, anguished, depressed or just evil, we must all protect ourselves from taking on other peoples emotions and problems. I was so grateful for his tenderness and compassion. He helped ease me out of my condition and by that night

I was almost back to normal.

I know the dangers of being overly empathetic. I know the concept of boundaries and the personal bubbles. But, my deep desire to help, overpowered my knowledge and good sense. One of my basic beliefs is based on airplane procedures, when the oxygen masks drop out from the ceiling, you must put your mask on first. If you don't take care of yourself, you can't help anyone else.

Since that episode with Maureen, I am very careful to keep my personal space protected and clearly defined. Remember the bubble boy? He was a little boy that had no immune system, so he had to live in a protected plastic bubble. I now work like the bubble boy, except that instead of a bubble made of plastic, mine is a spiritual bubble, all around me.

We should all maintain a personal bubble, an area of personal space around us, where we draw our boundaries. We are all energetic beings and there are some people that can suck our energy from us. You know who they are, they may be negative, or disgruntled, or always blaming others for their situation. Sometimes people who are unhappy can make you unhappy too. Guard against being drawn into someone else problems or anger. Try using an imaginary bubble.

I need to help people, that is my calling, but I must protect myself too, or I'm worthless at my job.

Maureen continued to come to me for help and I helped her as much as I could. I could adjust her entire spine and she always felt better when she left.

I still desperately wish that I could help her more, but I must trust that destiny has a hand in all things, and I'm no match for that.

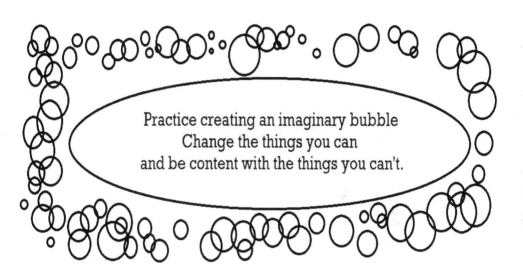

Practice creating an imaginary bubble
Change the things you can
and be content with the things you can't.

Chapter 23
Drugs, booze, and whores

At two years old, Young Georgie developed asthma. His mom brought him everywhere, andto everyone, looking for help. The medical doctors prescribed him drugs that his mother shoved down his throat. When that didn't work they restricted his diet, and then, she could only shove certain things down his throat. None of it did any good.

His father abandoned the family when George was only two years old. In that same year, little Georgie took a tumble down the post office steps. Sometime, during all that drama, Georgie developed asthma. Nothing anyone prescribed, or did, seemed to help Georgie with his life threatening condition. His mother had originally thought that he was acting up because his daddy was gone. Unfortunately, she had no sympathy for that. At first, she was harsh with him pushing him to toughen up. When it became clear that at times he was gasping for air, and had to be brought to the emergency room, she started to realize that it was more serious than just disappointment. She knew there was something wrong. Luckily for George, she was determined to fix it.

Years went by, and his mom had taken him everywhere, with no relief. One day while out shopping, she heard from some friends about a group of chiropractors that had worked wonders with one of their kids. Desperate for a cure, his mom, once again, drug him off to yet another Voodoo clinic. Back then, chiropractors were thought of as quacks. In some places, they still are. Georgie was her only child, if a chiropractor could help Geroge, she didn't care what he was.

Chiropractic used to be illegal, and history shows that we were imprisoned for helping people. In 1966, The American Medical Association, (AMA) advised its members that it was unethical for medical doctors to associate or refer patients to chiropractors. Nearly two decades later, in 1987, the AMA was found guilty of engaging in unreasonable restraint of trade and of conspiracy. The verdict put some federal restraints on the AMA's battle against chiropractors. But, even as late as 1965, not all states had made chiropractic legal and to recommend such a therapy was impossible for the regular medical doctor, and rare for the laymen.

With great anticipation, George was taken to the chiropractic clinic that was operating in a old Victorian mansion at the edge of town. The miracle worker, Dr. Lindquist D.C., was a big Swedish guy, whose whole family worked with him in his office. They offered chiropractic and Swedish massage, along with nutritional guidance and herbal remedies.

His condition had left Georgie, small for his age. So, his mother pushed her skinny, little runt of a son, into the office. Georgie was shaking with fear. The house was huge, the room was huge, and the Doctor was huge. Georgie was already shy to begin with, and when the doctor spoke to him, he was unable to speak. No matter, his mother usually spoke for him, anyway "Sit down and do what the doctor tells you" she said. The chiropractor took x-rays, and examined him thoroughly. After hours of careful study, he decided that the problem was in the area between the base of the skull and the first cervical vertebrae, called the sub-occipital space.

To this day, George remembers vividly, how the burly man took his scrawny neck into his large beefy hands, and cracked him. The crack was so loud, it was like a gunshot in his head. His mothers eyes popped open in astonishment, and he recalls the shocked look on her face. Seeing his mother's face, frightened him more than the cracking of his neck. George was left to lie quietly on the table, until things calmed down, and then, George was sent home with his mom to recuperate.

He said it was immediate. He could immediately feel the pressure lift off of his chest, and his breathing dramatically improved. He felt more alive. Puny until that point, his life changed that day. More and more robust, as the days passed, he never had trouble with his asthma again. The chiropractor asked his mom if he had taken any hard falls, but at the time, she couldn't remember anything. When she got home she remembered that day, five years ago, when little George had tumbled down the concrete steps of the post office. His asthma and the rest of his problems seemed to start some time after that.

After the adjustment, his appetite came back and his complexion changed from slightly gray to radiant pink. His mother continued to take him to the chiropractor throughout his childhood. In her eyes the doctor had performed a miracle. After that, whenever Georgie got sick or hurt, she took him to the chiropractor.

His single mother and his new stepfather were loving, but suffocating parents, and when George turned eighteen, he took off running head first as far away as he could get. Always a hard worker, his mother would tolerate no less, he had saved his money, so that he could leave home and go to college. He was successful at anything he tried. Studying chemistry and engineering, he and his buddies quickly set up a still in the frat house. They made beer and booze, thus, making them a popular bunch.

After he graduated, he changed jobs as often as he changed wives. He had several careers before he finally settled down as a water system inspector. He continued to visit the chiropractor, faithfully, all his life. I am his latest chiropractor, and he's been my patient and friend for the last seventeen years.

Always a ladies man, he's been married five times. Whenever his bride starts to tell him what to do, or tries to boss him around, the marriage disintegrates and George moves on. Even talking about someone trying to tell him what to do, makes him angry. As his doctor, I have regal status, because of my title, he will tolerate my strong suggestions for his health and welfare. He won't always follow my directions, but he doesn't get mad at me for bossiness and nagging.

At seventy five, he is alone and lonely. When a pretty girl walks by, he acts like a kid. He loves women and makes no attempt to hide it. He's not aggressive or rude. He's just smitten. Girls half his age, find a sympathetic listener, and a wise counselor in our George. George would like more, but he'll take what he can get, and he is patient. Like they say, even a blind squirrel finds a nut once in a while. Occasionally, George is rewarded with romance.

He lives in a retirement community that forbids drugs and alcohol. We know that George hates being told what to do, but he's also frugal. He goes along with it because the rent is really cheap. The discounted rent comes in exchange for putting restrictions on his life. The deal is, no drinking, no smoking, no drugs (that includes pot) on the grounds, or anywhere, even in the confines of your own unit.

George appears to go along with it, but he really doesn't. He likes drinking and smoking pot. He drinks and smokes regularly, but really no one's the wiser, as long as he's discreet. His unit is for single people only. After five divorces, George is content with being single.

Before he moved to his present digs, we had a mutual friend, Peter, who lived with George. He was a doctor, and was also bipolar. Peter was on prescription meds for his condition, but he hated taking his pills. Occasionally, and without warning, he would just stop taking them. It always ended badly. He'd end up in the hospital or on the floor. Without his meds he was a wreck and couldn't cope.

Last Fourth of July, our friend, Peter, dressed up in his own personal, amazing clown suit, performed in the parade. He marched down Main Street with his big floppy clown shoes and a red nose. We all sat on the sidelines, laughing and clapping, as he danced and skipped, merrily down through the center of town. That was a good day; he had been taking his pills.

Not long after that fun, exciting day, Peter, once again, stopped taking his meds. He drove his car into the woods, put one end of a hose in his exhaust pipe, and threaded the other end of the hose through the car window. Then he closed the windows and started the car. Letting the exhaust fill the car, he passed out and died. Devastated and shocked, we all wondered what we could have done differently. But, there was nothing we could do. He was off his pills. That was a bad day.

The episode with Peter didn't help George's drinking problem one bit. George was hiding in his cabin, drinking himself silly, and ignoring his friends. Although he never needed an excuse to drink, too often, and too much, this time George was over doing it, even for him. Peter's suicide got us all needing a drink.

And then, one morning, way too early for a casual call, I got a call from George. I didn't know who it was at first, but with six kids, when the phone rings, in the very late or very early hours, I jump and grab it. That morning, still between my sheets, I grabbed the phone, and half asleep, I blurted out into the receiver, "What?! What's wrong?!" I was fearful of the worst.

Well, the worst had happened for George. He had been drinking a little too much. Trying to walk into the bedroom he swayed, fell over sideways into the coffee table, we think, and then hit the floor. He regained consciousness some time in the night and realized that he couldn't move. Everything hurt. Luckily, he had the sense to shake the coffee table until his phone slid off onto the floor, where he could grab it. He called emergency, 911, for an ambulance. They put him on a stretcher and took him to the hospital. He, besides hitting his hard head, hard, had broken his leg. Not a good thing for a seventy five year old man.

The problem he was calling me about, was that George had a sweet little schnauzer named Stella. She would need to be taken care of while he was in the hospital. He knew Sheila, one of his prettier neighbors, would agree to go over to take care of her, but he couldn't have her going into his place until the booze, the drugs and the whores, had been cleared out. So he was calling me, his nefarious friend, to high tail it over there, and make the place look presentable. Meaning 'hide the evidence'.

Of course, I said yes. I love a good harmless caper. I only agreed with the understanding that if I needed help with something equally wicked, no matter how illegal or dangerous, he would help me with it, no matter what. I had him over a barrel, so he agreed. He was desperate. Who else would do such a thing for him without giving him away? Only a true and loyal, wild and crazy friend...Me!

Dragging myself out of bed, half asleep, I threw a jacket over my pajamas, drove over, found his key and let myself in. The place was a wreck, his little dog was barking her head off, and either she, or George, had knocked empty wine bottles and ashtrays onto the floor. The booze was all over the kitchen counter. Another glass had spilled onto the floor. The skunk weed could be smelled a mile away. There were no whores around, but who knows whether they were really there or not. Packing up all the evidence, I gave the dog a pet, locked up the house, and headed out to my car.

I started to back out, just as a motorcycle pulled into the driveway, and stopped right behind my car, blocking my exit. Under the helmet and black leathers was a lovely lady looking sternly at me. I had a feeling that I was looking at the most recent lover, or the gestapo. I stashed the bottle, the bag and the pipe, behind the seat of my car. Walking up to the car, she leaned into my window and asked, "what are *you* doing here?"

I'm glad I wasn't the other woman or she would have scared the snot out of me.

"I'm George's chiropractor" I said, "George has had an accident and is in the hospital. He called me this morning and asked me to get his wallet ." "I think he's gonna be okay but he needs someone to take care of the dog."

Taking off her helmet, she shook the kinks out of her hair, and said " Well, that's not me."

I smiled like a Cheshire cat. That old coot had latched onto a hottie. I was just certain that the smell of the skunk weed was wafting out my car, making me seem like a stoner. I hated having her think that, but I couldn't say anything without giving George away. She didn't look like an innocent neighbor, but I couldn't be sure. So smiling like a stooge, trying to look innocent, I made it clear that I was not George's lover.

"Tell Georgie that Gloria said Hi." she said, as she left.

Walking to the back of my car, she got on her Harley, and rode away. I bet she could tell George what to do, without him getting mad. I bet he liked it.

Breaking your leg at an advanced age is never good. But luckily, George wasn't frail, just drunk. His medical doctor was pretty sure booze was involved and wanted to know just how bad his problem was. George assured him that he was truly done with it all. So happy to be alive and still have his place to live, he swore off the booze.

Of course, the memories fade, when the worst is over. George began drinking again, but much more carefully and moderately.

"I don't want to tell you what to do," I told him, "but if you're gonna drink, you should get an alert button. What would have happened if you couldn't get to your phone? You could have died there. The lady in black might have showed up in time to save your life, but you can't count on that.

George listened in silence, "one other thing," I said, "you should be taking milk thistle, or sylmarin. It helps the liver clear out the alcohol and prevents hangovers." George is my friend if he is going to make bad choices, I can at least help him make the best of it.

When he comes in for his appointments, we warm up his body, stretch his muscles and talk about his mother and his ex-wives. We laugh about his love life, and we talk about which of his many older friends have died and, of course, I mention his need to curb his drinking and drug use.

At seventy five years old, curbing his bad behavior is a lesson in futility. Also at seventy five, he's lucky to be alive, so if it were me, I'd do whatever the heck I want.

George has spent his whole life fighting against people telling him what to do. I know the feeling. As an intelligent female, men have treated me like an idiot. They just naturally think that they know better and don't even consider my intelligence. I hate it. I understand that George hates it too. He's less adamant about it now, but why should anyone tell someone else how to live their life anyway.

Everybody has one life to live. You're not allowed to live another person's life for them. That's not fair. Even if you think you know better. You have yours, and I have mine.

I hope I never to have to clean up a mess or a murder, but if I do, I can always call George.

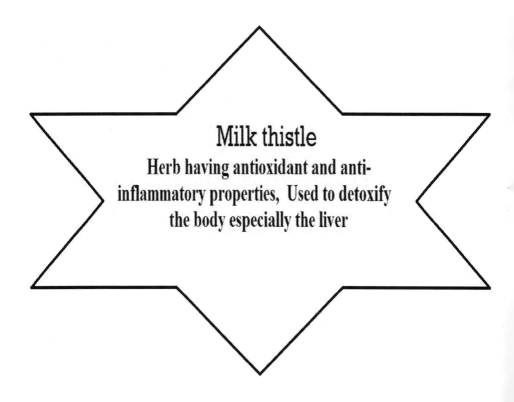

Milk thistle
Herb having antioxidant and anti-inflammatory properties, Used to detoxify the body especially the liver

Chapter 24
Pajama party

Leticia was very young when her parents, first took her to the doctor, to have her head examined. All her young life, she had suffered from migraines. They took skull X-rays and performed an EEG, searching for a reason why such a young girl, would have such horrible headaches. Their conclusion, after all the tests,was that she was nervous. She was twelve years old, and a nervous wreck. Her family life was fractious and unstable. Frightened in her own home, she was insecure and shy. She tried to hide and be quiet, knowing that if no one could see her, no one would hurt her. Her father was a drunk, and her mother was a screamer.

She took every new migraine drug, as it became available, but nothing worked. Her headaches continued throughout her life, and then, at the age of thirty seven, she decided to try a chiropractor.

Through the years, I've discovered that migraines respond extremely well to a sub-occipital lift. Its probably the same adjustment that the big Swedish chiropractor used to help George with his asthma. The sub-occipital area is a high traffic area for nerves and arteries. The very important vagus nerve passes through this narrow area. The vagus nerve is part of the autonomic nervous system known as the parasympathetic system. It commands and is responsible for an array of important body functions including: breathing, heart rate, blood pressure and digestion, among others. Doctors stimulate this cranial nerve to treat people with epilepsy or severe depression.

The first time I saw Leticia, I could feel the base of her skull was very congested. As she told me her story, I could see the little girl hidden beneath the skin of the woman who sat in front of me. My fingers were itching to do their work, and decompress that neck of hers. Laying on my table, she was hopeful, yet anxious. I imagine she thought, "what is this weirdo doctor going to do to me now" It's an unusual adjustment, so I try to prepare the patient by explanation and education.

Accidental traumas, like bicycle accidents, whiplash, diving headfirst into shallow water, birth injuries, especially forceps births, or simply falling can cause pinching and compression of the sub-occipital region. This untreated consdition can cause lifelong problems of headaches, vertigo, heart palpitations, high blood pressure, and digestive problems.

The best time to seek help with a migraine is when the migraine is in the initial stage of pre-syndrome, called an aura. A migraine aura usually occurs before the migraine actually strikes. Not everybody gets an aura before a migraine, but when they do, it is usually a visual disturbances, like seeing spots or lights, and can sometimes cause tingling or numbness in the face or arms. Once the migraine has reached it's full force, the adjustment isn't as effective.

The occipital lift has given countless patients relief. Donna is another migraine victim. She has on more than one occasion, desperate for relief, come stumbling into my office, dressed in pajamas, and cradling her vomit bowl.

Performing an occipital lift on Leticia, was like fireworks in my office. I usually hear a little crack, but with Leticia, it was multiple pops. Several levels in her neck had been compressed, and they all opened up that day. She said even her sinuses opened up and she felt like a weight was lifted from her shoulders. Leticia comes to my office whenever she gets a migraine aura. This sub-occipital adjustment helps relieve the pain and duration of the headache. It's also useful when patients are suffering from ear aches and sinus congestion, because the decompression allows the head to drain.

The last time she had a headache, I was out of town, (yes, again) and she was in severe blinding pain for several days. When her suffering finally faded, she was left with what is called a floater. A blurry blob that floats around in the line of vision, an unwanted residual effect from her migraine.

When I got back to my office, I gave her an occipital lift, and the floater disappeared.

Tension in the neck and shoulders, compresses the spine, nerves and sub-occipital space. This compression can initiates the migraine syndrome. Meditation and relaxation techniques, along with avoidance of personal triggers, can help reduce the incidence of migraines.   Triggers are different for different people, they can be emotional, physical exertion, or food triggers. Pleasantly hiking in the woods or sitting in the park can help to reduce the strain of life and boost the bodies production of DHEA, the hormone of eternal youth.

Psychotherapy, counseling, exercise or meditation can help relieve the underlying nervous tension. Herbal remedies with echinacea as a tonic, and tumeric for inflammation, if taken everyday, can help balance us.   Valerian root, hops, and passionflower, can also be used as muscle and nervous system relaxers.   I recommend that migraine sufferers do all of the above.

Chapter 25
Let's go dancing

Not every scrape and bruise has an emotional component to explore and expunge. When a medical situation arises, getting a second opinion is the wise path. Why not try the second opinion of a Chiropractor or mind body medicine worker. It certainly won't hurt to explore a different option.

Sometimes, a chiropractor can alleviate the pain that you were scheduled to fix through surgery. Like Roberta, whose rib pain led her to remove her gall bladder. Or Kelly, whose Lumbar vertebrae were causing leaky gut and neurological symptoms, mimicking Multiple Sclerosis. Or Donna, who enlisted the services of her husband and friends to get her to the chiropractor, for an occipital lift and migraine relief.

Drugs and surgery are not the only answer, and often not the best answer. Many times the problems originate in our hearts, souls, or minds.

I would just like to say that I would have finished this project sooner, but I needed to do some serious thinking. Yes, I am on the horns of a dilemma, and I just needed some quiet time, to meditate and consider.

So real time, Dr. Bluefish is going through real, life changing lessons. I am watching younger women do, what I have done years ago, and coincidentally, am doing again right now.   It's true that life is a spiral, We go round and round, circling at a little higher level each time, at least we hope. Life isn't over just because we're old or tired.   We learn the lessons of life, by bravely going deeper into the truth, with every turn of the screw.

I've decided to go out dancing and leave my problems at home, for now.   Once again, I feel blessed that there are places in this town where I can go out and be among friends. It's a bold decision to break out from   under my burden, let the consequences be damned, and head out into the night alone. I must not let fear dictate my choices, or rule my heart. Like my friend young Rachel is doing, I'm sticking up for myself! I need to put on *my* oxygen mask, first. I **need** to go dance!!

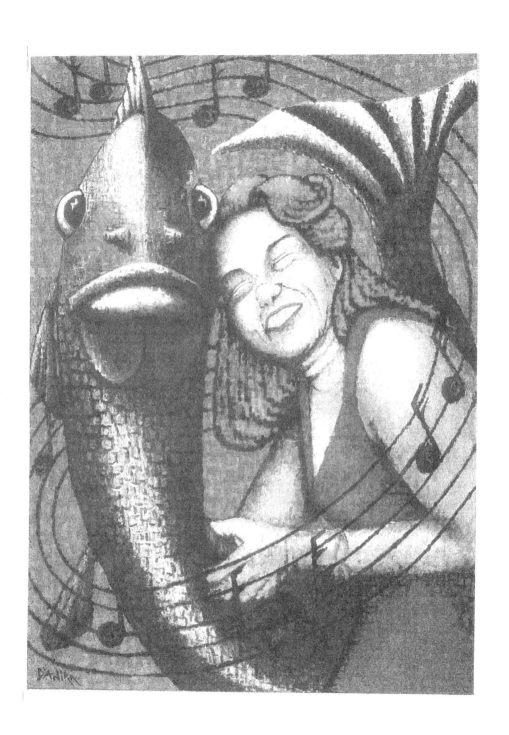

Bluefish and Mr. Right.

ABOUT THE AUTHOR

As a young child, I learned what it felt like to be in emotional and physical pain. There are advantages to a challenging childhood. Empathy and compassion are the primary benefits that come to mind.

My compassionate nature has always guided me in my journey to care for creatures, large and small. I started walking on my brothers back to ease his pain when I was five years old. I have always wanted to help everyone and everything.

I spent fifteen years of my life as a Registered Animal Health Technician. Working in animal hospitals in New Jersey, Oregon, and California, as well as in Emergency Clinics in those same states, I worked earnestly, compassionately and intuitively. Nursing, Radiology, Laboratory work, and surgical assisting were all included in my job description. I loved every minute of it.

After receiving some counseling for my struggling marriage I discovered that I could do so much more with my life.

At the age of thirty eight, I decided to go back to school to fulfill my dream of helping people feel better and regain health and longevity. As a wife and mother, it comes naturally to me to listen, and to advise. My difficult youth prepared me for solving problems not just for myself but for others. I am empathetic, meaning, I immediately feel the emotions emanating from people in my presence. I am a compassionate listener. People seem comfortable confiding in me and with our gentle sharing of stories and lessons, I seem to be able to help people transform their confusion into organization and their darkness into light. Deciding to become a doctor was one of the best decisions that I have ever made. Once again, I love every minute of it.

In my twenty years working as a chiropractic practitioner of mind body medicine, I have witnessed unusual and interesting stories of personal grief and growth. I earned a degree in Biology, Summa Cum Laude, from Fairleigh Dickinson University in New Jersey and a profession degree as a Doctor Of Chiropractic, Magna Cum Laude, from the Cleveland Chiropractic College in Hollywood, California. I have drawn from years of education and my many years of experience in my practice and in my personal life to come to my conclusions with accompanying advise and guidance.

I joined Mensa the high IQ society when I realized from academic testing that, although I have always felt like a freak, it was not because I was stupid, like I had been told, but because I was smarter than the average bear. My life has been spent helping all creatures, animals and people, regain health and longevity.

This book is a compilation of gossip and mind body treasures. When presented with a patient struggling with common and uncommon personal problems, I use these true stories to illustrate possible roads to self realization and recovery. The science and philosophy contained in these tales provides insight into what others, who have had the same problems, have learned and what they have done to help themselves. I include the strangest, along with the most common stories, I have heard and include the self help wisdom and advice used successfully to recover balance and health.

I present here my favorite poem. The one that sums it all up.

For Whom The Bell Tolls
No man is an island,
Entire of itself,
Every man is a piece of the continent,
A part of the main.
If a clod be washed away by the sea,
Europe is the less.
As well as if a promontory were.
As well as if a manor of thy friend's
Or of thine own were:
Any man's death diminishes me,
Because I am involved in mankind,
And therefore never send to know for whom the bell tolls;
It tolls for thee.

John Donne

I would like to give *Special Thanks* to
Rebecca Amber Davis Moyers

AUTHORS WEBSITE
drbluefish.com

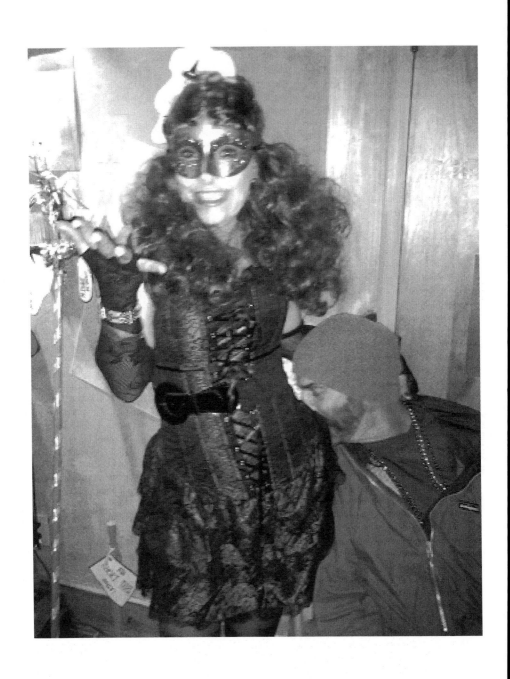

Cest Fini !

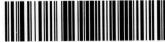

Made in the USA
Columbia, SC
28 March 2018